baby and you

The Real Life Guide to Birth and Babies

Compiled by Rosalyn Thiro

with contributions from Robin Barker, Kate Figes,
Jane Hobden, Sheila Kitzinger and others

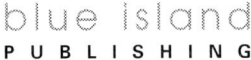

baby and you

First published
in 2002 by
Blue Island Publishing
Aberdeen House,
22–24 Highbury Grove
London N5 2EA

www.blueisland.co.uk

Compilation © 2002
Rosalyn Thiro

ISBN 0-9540802-1-1

No part of this
publication may be
reproduced, stored in
a retrieval system, or
transmitted in any
form or by any means,
electronic, mechanical,
photocopying,
recording or
otherwise, without
the prior written
permission of the
copyright owner.

Printed and bound
in England by
Mackays of Chatham

Distributed by
Central Books
99 Wallis Road
London E9 5LN

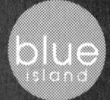

CONTENTS

4 INTRODUCTION

7 THE LONG MONTHS OF PREGNANCY

37 THE HOURS OF LABOUR

59 THE FIRST DAYS TOGETHER

77 BABYCARE CONTEXTS

111 A BIG CHAPTER ABOUT FEEDING

153 A BIG CHAPTER ABOUT SLEEP

199 LOVE AND TRIUMPH

215 THE REST OF LIFE

A Note From the Editor

This book is about having a baby in the real, modern world.

As the compiler, editor and principal author of this book, I thought it would be useful to bring together the most important topics relating to pregnancy, birth, babycare and motherhood in one volume. I had the idea for this about two months after having a baby myself (a lovely, longed-for little girl in the summer of 2000). Like many other mothers-to-be, I had attended labour and breastfeeding classes, and read a range of books. Not having had much experience with babies in the past, I was willing to learn from any source available. But contradictions became increasingly apparent in what I was hearing and reading. The most obvious areas of contention seemed to be between natural or medicalised birth, breast or bottle feeding, getting inoculations or not, going back to work or not. The innocent-looking childcare manuals turned out to be pushing their own ideologies, many of them alluding to different bodies of medical or psychological studies to support the superiority of their methods. I was distracted by conflicting directives about how to relate to my child. Was I supposed to bring her into my bed or let her cry herself to sleep in a cot? To treat colic as a digestive disorder or a symptom of overtiredness? To feed her on demand or impose a feeding schedule? And so on.

From what I could observe in myself and many other new mothers I was meeting, all of us were feeling both ecstatic and vulnerable, developing our own ways of doing things, compromising on previously held ideals, understanding more about the issues at stake and forming opinions about every matter relating to babies. From absolute beginners, nervous about holding our own newborn infants, we were all becoming baby experts in our own right.

Having a baby is more all-consuming than most people imagine until they experience it for themselves. The difference between idealism and reality stems partly from what we are taught about birth and babies nowadays. The books and formal classes focus so much on clinical aspects (e.g. the stages of labour, the nutritive superiority of breastmilk, how to change a nappy and bath a baby etc) that the real nature of life with a new baby – an intense physiological and emotional relationship between mother and child – is somehow lost or diluted. Compounding the problem is the fact that there has been so much politicisation of birth, breastfeeding and sleep in recent years that first-time parents are often confused by the contradictory views and advice from different experts.

In the meantime, there is little hard practical advice given to new mothers about how the child's pattern of sleep will mature in the early months, and how to encourage the sleep cycles into a 24-hour rhythm, yet this is one of the most significant parts of the child's life and crucial to the parents. For example, I have heard in parentcraft classes and read in several babycare books such cursory and flippant comments as "sleep when the baby sleeps" or "you will learn to live with less sleep". Some people do adjust to broken sleep with relative ease, but chronic tiredness is also a well-known trigger for depression. I suffered insomnia as well as broken sleep in the early weeks of motherhood, which was a residue of a prolonged stay in an understaffed London maternity unit. I didn't sink into depression (I was otherwise well supported by others and delighted with motherhood), but I could appreciate how the stresses of fatigue and other factors might easily lead down that road. I began to research the area of sleep and other issues relating to the new mother's situation.

At five months, when my insomnia was fading, I started contacting some of the movers and shakers in the political world of babies, inviting them to contribute. I also sent questionnaires to 20 new mothers, asking them to write about their experiences of British maternity facilities, labour, breastfeeding, sleep, bonding, going back to work and other topics. Contrasting stories and anecdotes began to flood in from these women and another 30 parents, with whom I kept in correspondence as they lived through the precious first years after childbirth. My own stories are amongst those that appear in the book.

What follows is a compilation of the most important issues and practicalities, as I see them, that British women face in the journey from pregnancy through the early months of parenthood. The book focuses mainly on the experiences of mothers, not because fathers don't count, but because it is women who come under far more social pressures as well as the physical duress of child-bearing and breastfeeding. Most sections are written by me; others, where indicated, are written by Sheila Kitzinger, Kate Figes, Robin Barker, Jane Hobden and experts from the midwifery profession and other authorities. (See pp238–239 for more information about these experts and the 50 parents who contributed.)

In the course of compiling the book, I have also concluded that most literature on babycare is much more polarised into "child-centred" approaches or "rules and regimes" than is reflected by what we do in real life. There is a middle way between imposing a regime on your baby or always following your baby's lead, which becomes blindingly obvious when you speak with other families and find your own way through daily life as a parent. We all build up our own ideologies in relation to parenthood: the broad middle way is my own, and I have included a middle-way sleep strategy, based on advice from sleep experts, amongst other practical suggestions. I also believe that babycare itself cannot be separated from the way you feel towards your child – your altered sense of self, deepening love, possessiveness and even morbid fears will all have a bearing on how you go about parenting. Therefore, I challenge the majority of child-centred teachings, which leave out the parents' emotions and needs in their ideologies.

My hope is that other new mothers will find the book helpful, both in the practicalities of birth and babycare, and for understanding the political context of what they read and hear from other sources. I also hope that amongst the selected stories you will find a genuine sense of empathy to resonate with your own experience of having a baby.

Rosalyn Thiro

Comments about this book are welcome
email info@blueisland.co.uk

THE LONG MONTHS OF PREGNANCY

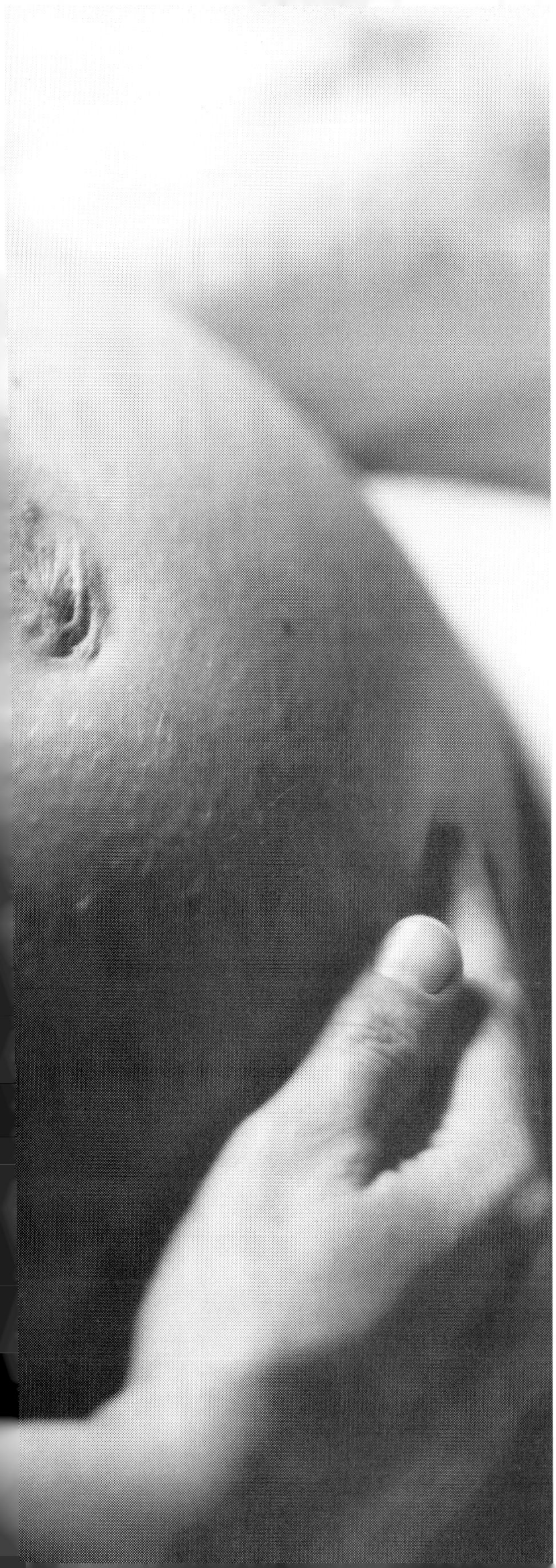

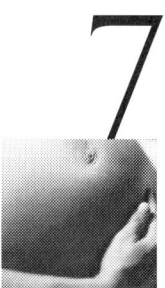

Contents

8   Excitement and Secret Fears

12   Maternity Facilities

16   What We Learn During Pregnancy

20   Interventions and the Midwife Crisis

28   Birth Politics

32   Views on Birth Politics

Excitement and Secret Fears

The word "pregnant" derives from the Latin for "before birth", suggestive of a mysterious time without definite beginning. With ultrasound and illustrations of the growing foetus, the time before birth has now lost some of its mysteries. Yet such knowledge does not diminish the secret thrills and worries of pregnancy.

Life in the Balance

Many pregnancy manuals illustrate the different stages of the growing foetus and give advice about all aspects of maternal and foetal health, from morning sickness to placenta praevia. They do it very well, and this book does not attempt to compete with them. Instead, the editor wants to look at pregnancy as the start of a monumental relationship, with all its attendant hopes, worries and life-changing assaults upon the sense of self. Looking through various dictionaries, the other meanings of the word "pregnant" tellingly show a torrent of concepts such as "momentous", "imaginative", "teeming" and even "threatening".

A first pregnancy is a time of transition and also a state of body and mind unto itself. It is often viewed as a time of security, the purest bond between mother and child. Yet, if there's one thing that's perhaps universal to first-time mothers-to-be, it's an underlying doubt that their pregnancy can really culminate in a live, healthy baby. Such doubt is not surprising given the struggle for life that takes place in the womb. Estimates suggest that about one in three humans die before the third month *in utero*. Of babies who make it to three months, the risks decrease dramatically. Only one or two in a hundred will die at a later stage of gestation. From knowing such odds, many women try to suppress feelings of excitement during the first trimester. The 12-week scan now takes on more significance than the emerging sensation of movements ("quickening") at four to five months, which was the main milestone of pregnancy for countless generations before us. Ideas about early bonding are covered on pp200–202.

Women who have miscarried in the past often become suspicious of their own bodies. They dare not assume that this pregnancy will be "the one". Even when pregnancy is well established and the main time of danger is past, some nagging doubt can hold you back from enjoying your pregnancy. When people offer congratulations, you almost wish they wouldn't lest ultimately there is nothing to celebrate. The editor and several other women interviewed for this book felt like this for at least the first half of pregnancy, if not the whole of it.

A first pregnancy can take an age. At 20 weeks you cannot believe you are only halfway; at 32 weeks, the thought of being 40 weeks can seem both remote ("will I feel different then?") and all too close ("I'm not prepared for this"). Birth is a massive psychological hurdle; the time beyond birth virtually unimaginable. Meanwhile, feeling your breasts and belly swell and your baby moving within are the most peculiar, secret thrills.

Often, if we divulge our secret worries to others – such as friends or health professionals – we are told "don't worry" or "that's a normal worry". Obviously, it's not a good situation if the negative emotions predominate during pregnancy, but such feelings should not necessarily be suppressed or dismissed *per se*. In some ways, it can be more positive to view pregnancy as a time when life is in the balance. There are no certainties with anything relating to babies. Once you get through one worry, another one will probably rise up in its place – what a scan might reveal; what might happen in labour; inoculations; touching a plug socket; climbing a tree. We are concerned about our offspring from the moment we learn of their existence up until the moment that we either learn of their demise or die ourselves, whether that is three weeks after conception or decades into the future. And this is perfectly ok – after all, concern, not indifference, is a basic feature in loving families.

Another, perhaps universal, fear is of having a child with an abnormality. Again, it's an understandable concern that shouldn't be belittled (the statistic for congenital conditions is 4% – see p74). Other worries might be about your relationship with the baby's father, your career, money, home. In your mind, birth might begin to take on the spectre of a gateway to either an island paradise or penitentiary. Love, happiness and life itself may all seem to hang in the balance, ready to take you on to new levels of joy or plunge you into despair. But this is a less positive way of viewing the situation, and unrealistic too. However your baby turns out and whatever your circumstances may be a year from now, life will likely be an indivisible mix of the highs and lows. In the words of one father interviewed, "it's the epiphanic inscribed in the goings-on of the everyday!"

The reason why speculation runs riot during the long months of pregnancy is because the baby is tucked away, silent and unseen. Of course, the pregnancy is a physical reality, placing demands on your body, but the baby is, psychologically, an abstract concept. At the same time, you can also feel a sense of contentment with your embraceable belly, lulling away worries for the time being...

Excitement and Secret Fears

Pregnancy Politics

During pregnancy is when you start to take on the mantle of parental and social responsibility. Not only do you have to make practical changes in lifestyle, but also you will probably become aware of other people scrutinising your actions. We are given directives about what we should and shouldn't do for the sake of our child's health. Most of us are generally happy to comply with these things because they feel like a proactive way of nurturing the little entity inside, who otherwise develops without intervention. But the advice is sometimes contradictory or so reduced to a sound bite ("avoid soft cheese") that the real risk factor is either lost or magnified in our minds. These are the main pregnancy politics:

Avoiding some foods We are told in countless sources to avoid mould-ripened and unpasteurised cheese, because of the risk of listeria, which is dangerous during pregnancy. But bear in mind that it's a tiny risk from these sources. On the other hand, salmonella is widespread in raw poultry and eggs, so cook these properly (as you would always). The popular brands of mayonnaise are fine because they use pasteurised egg. Toxins in shellfish are quite common, but illness is not inevitable. Liver can be packed with more vitamin A than is good for the foetus, but few people eat enough liver for this to be a risk.

There is absolutely no reason whatsoever to worry about having eaten one of the "banned" foods during early pregnancy if you didn't get ill. And even if you do get a stomach upset (as many women do during pregnancy, because nine months is a long time to go without some form of illness), it will not inevitably lead to miscarriage or abnormalities.

Cutting down on alcohol This is probably the most contentious of the pregnancy directives. Medical research has shown definite health risks of heavy drinking during pregnancy (foetal alcohol syndrome). The health authorities in the UK and many other countries regard "heavy" as five or six drinks a day (40 units a week). That kind of drinking is heavy enough to affect the adult's health and be called alcoholic.

Light alcohol intake – a top limit of ten units per week – is not regarded as a problem by the majority of health authorities. (A unit is a small glass of wine or half a pint of beer.) A small number of researchers have claimed that any alcohol can affect a child's future mental capacities, but such studies have not been considered rigorous enough to be accepted by the medical community at large. The UK's Health Education Authority currently states that "there is no evidence that light or occasional drinking in pregnancy will harm your baby". In France, women are apparently told to limit themselves to two or three glasses

THE LONG MONTHS OF PREGNANCY

of wine per day, and a Chinese doctor told the editor of this book that a little red wine each day would actually help the placenta. At the other end of the scale, pregnant women in the USA are so discouraged from drinking alcohol that in some States they can be arrested for doing so.

British women are supposedly becoming heavy social drinkers these days, so cutting down may be in order if you drink regularly. Binge drinking and getting drunk are obviously unwise, but if you are used to a wine or beer with food a few times a week, there's no need to stop, given the weight of research evidence so far. In fact, a lot of British women self-impose virtual abstinence from alcohol during pregnancy, especially if they miscarried in the past. Many of us have a nagging worry about alcohol intake before we discovered the pregnancy. It can help to know, however, that foetal alcohol syndrome is linked with heavy drinking during the second trimester, not the first. Miscarriage during the first trimester is common whether a woman drinks or not, so don't tear yourself apart worrying about what you drank. Some of us would not exist at all had our parents not been "under the influence" at conception.

Giving up smoking Unlike a light intake of alcohol, it seems from all the medical research to date that smoking of any kind is a very definite risk. Each time you inhale cigarette smoke, your baby's heart rate goes up, the newly formed lungs get a dose of nicotine and the placenta becomes a bit less efficient. The babies of women who smoke are more likely to be premature and suffer breathing problems. Smoking is linked to a greater risk of chest infections, asthma, coughs and cot death (see p196). Apparently, 20% of British women continue smoking – pregnancy, after all, is a stressful time. But, given all the other pregnancy directives aimed at us, is it clear that the risk to the child's health and life is thousands of times greater than eating a piece of Brie?

Taking it easy Being expected to take it easy can be an insidious form of pregnancy politics. If you feel relatively sprightly, there's no need to lie around for the sake of satisfying expectations. Indeed, the fitter your heart and lungs are, the better you will cope with the massive physical feat that is labour. On the other hand, if your body is screaming at you to slow down, then do so. To some women that will sound obvious, but to others it might mean compromising a resolution to carry on as normal in the face of having a baby.

Birth politics When pregnant, many of us become aware of the contention surrounding medical interventions during labour. This is a significant subject affecting maternity services, and is covered later in this chapter.

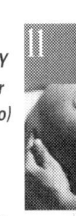

MOTHERS' BOOKS ABOUT PREGNANCY
• *Becoming a Mother* by Kate Mosse (Virago) is one of the few pregnancy books to look at different womens' experiences.

• *The Best Friend's Guide to Pregnancy* is a quirky take on the subject written by American mother Vicki Iovine.

• *The Rough Guide to Pregnancy and Birth* by Kaz Cooke is another upbeat work with cartoon illustrations.

See p17 for the pregnancy and birth experts.

Maternity Facilities

As pregnancy progresses, you'll think more about birth and make practical plans. Most British women (about 97%) give birth in an NHS hospital. However, in an attempt to escape the medicalised setting, some women are keen to have their babies at home or to seek out midwife-led facilities. Here, women's health writer **Jane Hobden** looks at the options.

NHS Hospitals

Maternity units in NHS hospitals fall into two types. Larger hospitals usually have a specialist unit led by a consultant obstetrician. They tend to have the most technologically advanced equipment and teams of experts at hand should any complications occur. Smaller cottage hospitals (low-tech units) may have a GP or midwife unit, where the woman stays under the care of a GP and the midwives who work in their practice. (See Who's Who in Maternity Services p15.) Women using these units are generally expected to have a straightforward delivery.

Many hospitals encourage women to make their own choices about labour, as far as possible given their facilities and individual policies. Some provide low-tech delivery rooms, where birth can take place in a more intimate, less medicalised setting. Most British hospitals now have a birthing pool, which can be used for pain relief during labour and sometimes for the delivery too. Delivery suites sometimes have birthing stools and other equipment which enable women to kneel, squat or stand, putting active birth principles into practice (see p17). Find out in advance what facilities your local hospital has – ask if you can tour the maternity wards, so that the environment doesn't come as a surprise on the day you give birth. Some low-tech items for labour, such as a TENS machine (see p56), can be hired if the hospital doesn't have them.

After the birth, most women are moved onto a maternity ward with their babies. Some hospitals also provide a few separate rooms – costs vary but are usually £30–£50 a night. For more about postnatal wards, see p62.

Most of us give birth in the local NHS hospital because we are referred there by our GP. Many of us are happy enough to comply with this – the hospital and/or maternity services may have a good reputation; it might be reassuring to have all forms of pain relief and emergency facilities on hand. First-time mothers often want the guidance and support offered by hospital midwives as they come to grips with breastfeeding and other aspects of babycare. Women with older children may want to rest and recuperate in hospital as a brief release from the pressures of home. There may also be medical reasons why a woman should have her baby in hospital under the care of a consultant, for example, diabetes or a heart or kidney condition which may place mother and baby at risk.

It is worth bearing in mind, though, that there might be other options in your area for giving birth. You might have a choice of hospitals, or the possibility of a home birth.

Home Births

Just over 2% of women in the UK give birth at home attended by the midwife. Although this is a fraction of the number giving birth in hospital, increasing numbers of women are expressing an interest in having a home birth these days, including first-time mothers. It has been argued that home births are unsafe, but research suggests that a home delivery is as safe as a hospital delivery for women who have straightforward pregnancies. You will probably be advised to opt for a hospital birth if complications are anticipated.

Giving birth in the familiar surroundings of your own home can be more comfortable than the impersonal environment of a hospital ward. Birthing pools can also be hired for home use (see panel). But if a complication develops whilst you are in labour, or if you want the pain relief of an epidural, then you will have to transfer to the nearest hospital. This is because certain interventions, such as caesareans or delivery by forceps or the ventouse cap, can only be performed by a doctor, while epidurals have to be administered by an anaesthetist. For more on interventions, see pp20–23.

On some occasions, women who planned a home birth are asked to go into hospital because too few midwives are available on the day (see the Midwife Crisis, p24). However, women do have the legal right to give birth at home, and midwives have a statutory duty to attend home births. Find out about transfer rates in your local area if you are planning a home birth, and try to stay mentally prepared for the possibility that you might have to transfer. Also see Birth Politics, pp28–35, and Births That Don't Go "To Plan" on p71.

Midwife-Led Services

Some women hire an independent midwife as a way of ensuring more continuity of care through pregnancy, labour and the first weeks with a new baby. The fee is usually around £2,500. Women hiring an independent midwife feel that they have more opportunity to build a strong, trusting relationship with

BIRTHING POOLS
Many hospitals now have a birthing pool. Of the women who use a pool, the majority spend part of their labour in it, and a minority will actually give birth in it. You will not be able to use one if you need constant monitoring.

Pools can also be hired for home use:

• Splashdown Water Birth Services
17 Wellington Terrace
Harrow-on-the-Hill
Middlesex
HA1 3EP
0870 444 4403
www.splashdown.org.uk

• Active Birth Centre
See p17

Maternity Facilities (Jane Hobden)

their midwife and to enjoy holistic, individualised care. All independent midwives have yearly supervisory visits and equipment checks, and are required to ensure that their clinical practice is up to date. Most women taking this route want a home birth. An independent midwife can also accompany you to any hospital (either NHS or private), though responsibility of care will probably pass to the consultant-led team once in the hospital.

Some NHS "cottage hospitals" offer midwife-led services. The Edgware Birth Centre in London offers a midwife-led, "home from home" birthing environment. It is open to women in Northwest London and elsewhere who have had a low-risk pregnancy and are anticipating a normal birth. More than half the babies are born in water. If complications arise, requiring, for instance, an instrumental delivery or a caesarian, women are transferred to a nearby hospital. There are also a handful of private midwife-led birth centres offering similar facilities but where a fee is payable – contact the Independent Midwives Association. For more on the politics of midwife-led versus consultant-led services, see pp23–27.

Private Hospitals

A small proportion of women (about 0.5%) have their babies delivered at a private maternity unit. There are only a few in the UK – the largest and best-known is the Portland (see panel), which has gained fame for being the place where celebrities go for an elective caesarian. The Hospital of St John and St Elizabeth has a more holistic ethos. There is also a private unit in Southampton – the Wessex Maternity Centre. These three have high-tech birth facilites and also all the facilities of a hotel (e.g. your own room, television, phone and laundry service). The Birth Centre near St George's Hospital in South London is a private low-tech midwife-led unit.

Note that the services of these maternity units are not available through private schemes run by companies such as BUPA. Most health insurance companies do not cover the cost of a normal labour, but will usually cover the cost of emergency medical care. Costs range from about £3,500 to £7,000 for a normal delivery. In the event of major complications, you might be transferred to the nearest NHS hospital.

A few NHS hospitals, such as St Mary's in London, have an option of private maternity facilities. This may be a full maternity unit plus private rooms on a separate wing, or women may be admitted as private patients to the hospital's main maternity unit but are then transferred to the private wing after the birth. Costs vary but on average are around £900 for a normal delivery and around £400 a night for staying in a private room.

PRIVATE FACILITIES

The Portland Hospital
205-209 Great Portland Street
London W1N
020 7580 4400
www.theportlandhospital.com

Hospital of St John and St Elizabeth
60 Grove End Road
London NW8
020 7286 5126

Wessex Maternity Centre
Mansbridge Road
West End
Southampton
Hants SO18 3HW
023 8046 4721

Lindo Wing
St Mary's Hospital
South Wharf Road
London W2 1NY
020 7886 1465

THE LONG MONTHS OF PREGNANCY

WHO'S WHO IN MATERNITY SERVICES

Midwives – nurses who are specially trained to look after mothers and babies during normal pregnancy, labour and after the birth. Many NHS midwives work with local GP practices providing antenatal and postnatal care as well as delivering babies in hospitals and at home. Some areas operate a team midwifery system for all antenatal care and the delivery. With another approach – known as the Domino Scheme – a midwife will come to see you at home when you go into labour, accompany you to hospital for the birth and then return home with you and the baby afterwards. Hospital midwives do shifts in the hospital's antenatal clinic and on the labour and postnatal wards, and some offer classes on labour, breastfeeding and perhaps water birth (see p16). A few maternity units are run by midwives rather than doctors – see previous page. For more on midwives, see pp24–26.

Obstetricians – doctors who specialise in the care of women during pregnancy, labour and the early postnatal period. In the hospital, you will be under the care of a consultant obstetrician's team of doctors and other health professionals such as midwives. Some women are referred to the consultant obstetrician during antenatal care. However, if you have a straightforward pregnancy and labour, you may not come into direct contact with your obstetrician at all.

Paediatricians – doctors specialising in the care of babies and children. A pediatrician may check your baby soon after the birth or, if labour has been difficult, might be asked to be present at the delivery.

Obstetric physiotherapists – trained to help women cope with the physical changes of pregnancy, childbirth and afterwards. Some run antenatal classes on relaxation and breathing, and exercises. After childbirth they advise on postnatal exercises and can check problems such as back strain.

Breastfeeding counsellors – some hospitals have a dedicated breastfeeding expert who can offer help and suggestions for women having difficulties either while they are in hospital or when they go home. Charity-supported breastfeeding counsellors also operate – see p130.

Health visitors – community-based nurses trained to look after the needs of the whole family. They take over postnatal care from midwives after about ten days. Your local health visitor will visit you at home initially, after which you can visit her at a child health clinic or the local practice depending on your area.

MIDWIFE-LED FACILITIES
Edgware Birth Centre (NHS)
Burnt Oak Broadway
Edgware
Middlesex
HA8 0DD
0208 732 6777
www.birthcentre.co.uk

Independent Midwives Association
1 The Great Quarry
Guildford
Surrey
GU1 3XN
01483 821104
www.independentmidwives.org.uk

Birth Centre (private)
37 Coverton Road
London SW17
020 7498 2322

What We Learn During Pregnancy

At the time when our grandmothers were pregnant, birth was a taboo subject, and there are stories of some women going into labour without much idea of what was happening. But how can a woman really prepare for her first labour and motherhood? **Jane Hobden** *looks at what we learn from formal classes and the experts during the long months of pregnancy.*

Midwife-Led Classes

NHS-run antenatal classes are popular, especially amongst first-time mothers-to-be. According to a 1998 survey across the general population, 40% of women attended antenatal classes, most of which were run by midwives. The classes, which are free, are held in hospitals and in local GP practices and health centres. They often take place during in the evening or at the weekend so you have the option of attending with your partner.

The sessions are mainly information and discussion-based, covering the main aspects of pregnancy and childbirth. Information is also given about the local hospital system, what happens when a woman is admitted to hospital, and the support available when she leaves. The classes provide an opportunity to meet midwives on the local team. Health visitors may attend some sessions in order to explain their role. Such classes can also be a good way of meeting other pregnant women and their partners. Some health authorities offer breastfeeding classes and "parentcraft", which might cover topics such as hygiene and first aid. Maternity units with birthing pools might offer a special class about water births.

The National Childbirth Trust

The National Childbirth Trust (NCT) is an independent organisation – members are mothers rather than medical professionals – providing a contrast to the more medicalised teachings about birth and also offering an alternative source of postnatal support. Across the country, over 15,000 women and couples a year attend fee-paying NCT antenatal classes. Such classes aim to cover all aspects of childbirth preparation, including what happens during labour and birth, the discussion of feelings, practical ways of coping with labour (including the role of the partner) and information about pain relief. Breastfeeding (which the NCT is

THE LONG MONTHS OF PREGNANCY

very keen on) and some aspects of babycare are also covered. Classes, which get booked up quickly, vary in length from intensive courses lasting a weekend to two-hourly sessions held weekly over eight weeks.

NCT classes clearly vary from area to area, and while many teachers give full, impartial information about different types of pain relief and common interventions during childbirth, some have been criticised for placing too much emphasis on natural childbirth and for implying that most women will have this type of birth. (See some of the anecdotes about classes on p19.) Whatever your personal thoughts on this, such classes can be a good way of meeting with others who are at a similar stage of pregnancy. There is usually a postnatal reunion, and group members are encouraged to keep in touch with each other.

ACTIVE BIRTH AND YOGA CLASSES

Another organisation running fee-paying antenatal classes is the Active Birth Centre. As the name implies, the Centre promotes a holistic approach to childbirth. The courses cover body awareness, relaxation and massage, and the role of the birth partner. A major part of the sessions is in identifying active ways of coping with labour – such as adopting deep breathing techniques, concentrating on making low noises or chanting to help ride contractions, and trying out different positions that go with gravity. It has been noted that class leaders often encourage women to question hospital practices, and there may be open criticism of the detrimental effects of standard medical interventions. There is a lot of support for water births and for giving birth at home rather than in hospital. The Centre has a commercial side, too, selling the Active Birth Ball (a prop for different positions) and massage oils.

Antenatal yoga classes are becoming increasingly popular. As well as providing a forum to help women keep fit and supple during pregnancy, the focus tends to be on relaxation techniques, body awareness and preparing the body for birth. Many of the classes offer refreshments after the exercise is over, providing an opportunity to get to know other pregnant women locally and to swap experiences and information.

WHAT THE BIRTH EXPERTS SAY

Sheila Kitzinger The best-known birth guru has been at the forefront of birth politics since the 1960s and is one of the contributors to this book – see p32. A social anthropologist, she has devoted much of her life to researching birth practices in different cultures (covered in *Rediscovering Birth*), and campaigning for more humane treatment of women in maternity hospitals, and for home birth. The *New Pregnancy and Childbirth* continues to be one of the most

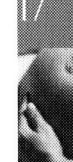

CLASSES
For NHS classes, speak to your midwife.

The National Childbirth Trust
Alexandra House
Oldham Terrace
Acton, London
W3 6NH
0870 444 8707
www.nctpregnancy andbabycare.com

Active Birth Centre
25 Bickerton Road
London
N19 5JT
020 7482 5554
www.activebirth centre.com

popular books with mothers-to-be, and it includes detail about alternative breathing techniques to try during labour. Sheila Kitzinger views labour as a psycho-sexual experience and firmly believes that the West can learn a lot from birth practices in traditional cultures, which do not disempower the labouring woman. She also offers the Birth Crisis Network for mothers who are experiencing post-traumatic stress disorder after a bad birth (for details see her web page www.sheilakitzinger.com).

Gordon Bourne His *Pregnancy* manual, first written in the 1970s, is still popular. He was an obstetrician and talks of "frequency of micturation" to describe how you might want to pee more often when pregnant. Some of his views are undeniably dated. Even in the revised edition, water births are dismissed as a fad. But if you are not into the ideas about active birth, and you don't mind that the advice is coming from a man, then his book is about as comprehensive as you can get for the clinical process of pregnancy and birth.

The What to Expect When You are Expecting book The authors are not particularly famous in their own right, but this is one of the most popular sources of information about pregnancy and birth, written with great deference to the American obstetric profession. They also have a babycare manual, see p83.

Janet Balaskas This is the birth guru who coined the term "active birth" and founded the Active Birth Centre in London as well as writing a number of books on the subject. She stresses the importance of being an active participant in your own pregnancy and birth, rather than a passive patient, and she draws analogies between contractions and ocean waves. She trained with the NCT.

Michel Odent A French obstetrician, Odent gained fame in the 1970s for introducing home-like birthing rooms to a state-run French hospital. He went on to found the Primal Health Research Centre in London, which studies the long-term effects of experiences in early childhood. He's also told fathers to stay away while the mother is in labour, contrary to the current trend of encouraging male participation in the birth event.

Do We Learn Enough During Pregnancy?

Most pregnant women are keen to learn as much as possible about birth and babycare. In a questionnaire sent to 20 new mothers, the editor asked for their views about what they learnt from formal classes. Touring the maternity unit and taking classes on labour and breastfeeding were mentioned by most as very

THE LONG MONTHS OF PREGNANCY

useful, but the general consensus was that there was not enough about the time after birth. As Julia said, "apart from breastfeeding, there was very little about caring for the baby – a big omission." Justine was also critical: "The first hospital antenatal class was just waffle about nothing. More focused classes were useful, though some midwives assumed we all had a lot of knowledge and asked us to "lead" the discussion." A few women mentioned that the formal classes came surprisingly late during pregnancy – well into the third trimester. Collette actually gave birth before she was due to do the midwife's class.

Of the women who had done NCT classes, the reaction was also mixed. Julia said that her partner gained a lot from knowing about different positions during labour, otherwise the classes had not been very useful. But Ruth had found the NCT classes helpful, "mostly because the woman holding them was excellent – not ideological, completely impartial and humorous. Otherwise, I read a few books and used the Internet, but quickly one assimilates the basics, and you start to find yourself reading the same information over again." Many couples could discern a distinct agenda from the NCT classes about fighting the medical system for the right to give birth with as little intervention as possible. This idea was reinforced by what they had read or heard about active birth. (The next sections of this book look at birth politics in more detail.)

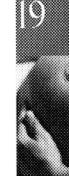

Several women had found antenatal yoga classes excellent for dealing with aches and pains in pregnancy, and breathing during labour. Some had not. Justine found that the most useful thing to come out of all her antenatal classes was anecdotal evidence and support, and subsequent postnatal friendships. "But I remember a couple of weeks before birth I started panicking about my lack of knowledge about caring for a baby."

Justine's "panic" is understandable. Basically, we learn very little about the time beyond birth while we are still pregnant. This is partly because birth is a vast psychological hurdle for the first-time mother-to-be. It isn't so surprising that few of us can bear to think in great detail about the time beyond when there may be a nagging doubt about whether there will be a baby at all at the other end of labour... It is also difficult to read the traditional childcare manuals while pregnant, because so many of them focus on the health aspects of babycare, which might seem irrelevant until a specific health query arises. Few formal classes cover anything relating to life with a baby other than breastfeeding. Labour and delivery are often discussed in terms of being the culmination of pregnancy more than as marking the start of parenthood, life's greatest challenge. It was partly from dissatisfaction with the formal NHS and NCT classes that the editor decided to compile this book...

Interventions and the Midwife Crisis

Medical intervention during labour is high and increasing in Western countries, a situation that has caused concern and attracted media attention. A complex issue for the obstetric profession, high intervention rates in the UK have also been linked by some researchers with a shortage of midwives in the NHS. **Jane Hobden** looks at the issue.

The Main Interventions

Medical interventions during labour are common. Nationwide figures show that 21% of women are induced, about a third have an epidural, general or spinal anaesthetic, and more than 20% have a caesarian. Listed below are the main types of intervention and some of the reasons behind the statistics.

Induction Labour is artificially induced if the health of mother or baby is deemed at risk. It is a common procedure with about one in five women being induced. Recommendations for induction might be if there is a worry that the baby is no longer receiving enough nutrition from the placenta (which might be the case if the baby is overdue), or if the mother's waters have broken without labour starting spontaneously within four days (or other duration according to hospital policy), as there is an increased risk of infection. Induction might also be strongly recommended if the mother has pre-eclampsia, high blood pressure, or some other condition, or if the baby no longer appears to be thriving in the womb.

Contractions are started by the introduction of synthetic hormones via an intravenous drip in the arm, or by inserting a pessary or gel into the vagina. Sometimes both methods are used and may be combined with rupturing of the membrane around the baby to release amniotic fluid. This is done using a small hook. The process may be a bit uncomfortable for you but is not painful or harmful to either you or the baby as there are no nerve endings in the membranes.

In some cases, it may take several attempts at induction over a number of hours or even days before labour is underway. Once it gets going, however, an induced labour can build up to intense contractions more quickly than when labour starts naturally. This means that the duration of labour might be relatively shorter, but the onset of pain harder to adjust to.

The Long Months of Pregnancy

According to guidelines from the National Institute for Clinical Excellence, women with trouble-free pregnancies should be offered induction if their pregnancy extends beyond 41 weeks as this reduces the risk of complications during labour, including the risk of stillbirth. However, as the Royal College of Midwives points out, women should be able to discuss whether induction is needed with their health professionals and the guideline should not override the woman's choice. It is calling for more research into the normal variation of the length of pregnancy and the effect of long gestation on mother and baby.

Episiotomy Women are given an episiotomy when the vaginal opening needs to be made bigger to allow the baby's head to pass through. Sometimes they are performed to speed up the birth because the baby is becoming short of oxygen. Carried out just before delivery, a local anaesthetic is given and the tissue of the perineum is then cut. Once the baby is born, the incision is sewn up with stitches which dissolve a few days later.

About 15% of women have an episiotomy during childbirth, often when forceps or ventouse are used (the rates are 80% and 65% respectively). However, the rate has been dropping since the early 1990s when the level was over 20%. This is partly because of the rise in caesarean sections (see p23), but also because it is now felt that episiotomies are sometimes unnecessary, and a minor tear can heal more quickly. With skilled guidance from midwives, more women now give birth without sustaining injury to the perineum.

Speeding up labour A woman's labour can be speeded up with an oxytocin drip which helps to strengthen uterine contractions. This may be used if your uterus is not working effectively or if contractions start to weaken during the course of a long, hard labour.

Epidural This is a powerful spinal anaesthetic used during labour, which has the effect of numbing the body from the waist down. It is injected into the outer membrane around the spinal cord through a fine tube. This is then left in place so that the anaesthetic can then be pumped in continuously or topped up when necessary. An epidural has to be administered by an anaesthetist, although it can be topped up by midwives. It usually takes about 20 minutes to site the tube and another 20 minutes for the anaesthetic to work. Epidurals are a very effective form of pain relief, and one in five of us opts for one. They are especially worthwhile for women who are having a prolonged or difficult labour, because they allow you to rest and perhaps even sleep for some hours

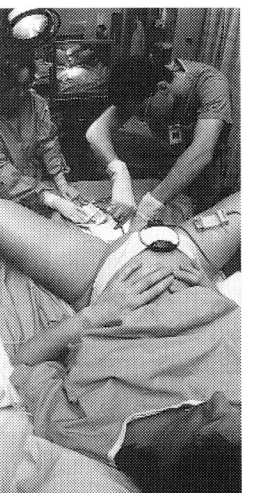

Obstetric monitoring and interventions such as episiotomy (below) make birth safer but can also leave you feeling like a laboratory animal.

Interventions and the Midwife Crisis

while your cervix continues to dilate. However, there are a number of major drawbacks with epidurals. Occasionally they only partially work – mainly due to the difficulty of injecting into the right place on your back. If you have one then you will probably be unable to get out of bed and may need a catheter to pass urine as well as a drip to provide fluids and help maintain blood pressure. (Some maternity units offer the option of a mobile epidural, which allows a woman to move her legs whilst providing an effective form of pain relief.) Oxytocin may also be needed to make the uterus work harder, and the baby will need to be monitored continuously.

Perhaps most significantly, the numbing effect of the epidural may mean that you have little urge to push once you have fully dilated. Furthermore, the natural tone of the pelvic floor muscles, which helps to rotate the baby's head, will be lost. Some women who have had an epidural do manage to push the baby out without help, especially if timing allows for the epidural to wear off for the pushing stage. Others need assistance with forceps or a vacuum cap. In some cases, a caesarian is needed to get the baby out. Because of this possibility of further interventions and because it can take some time to set up an epidural, you might be advised not to have one if you are nearly fully dilated at the time you crave relief. If this is the case with you, it can help to know that for the sake of a relatively short duration of continuing pain, you might be saving yourself from possible complications.

Forceps delivery or vacuum extraction About 10% of babies are delivered using either forceps or vacuum extraction (ventouse). After the mother is given a painkilling injection at the birth canal opening, the forceps – which look like a pair of salad servers – are placed around the baby's head and the baby is pulled along the birth canal. With vacuum extraction, a rubber cap attached to a suction device is fitted to the baby's head, which is then used to suck the baby out. Vacuum delivery tends to be used wherever possible instead of forceps, as there is evidence that there is less risk of damage to the birth canal and it is seen as a gentler form of birth for the baby. An episiotomy is often needed in both cases (see p21). Such methods of delivery are used when the second stage of labour has been prolonged, when the mother is exhausted, or when the baby is showing signs of distress and needs to born quickly.

Caesarian section The baby is delivered abdominally rather than vaginally. The incision is made through the abdomen and then the womb – the cut is usually crossways and just below the bikini line. The baby is then delivered, and the incision is sewn up. The whole operation takes about 40 minutes.

The Long Months of Pregnancy

If you have a caesarian then you will probably be given an epidural or spinal anaesthesia (which can be administered more quickly than an epidural), which means that you will remain conscious during the operation while your lower half is numb. A screen will be put across your chest so that you and your partner do not have to witness the operation. General anaesthesia (which is slightly more risky to the patient's health) is usually only used these days when a quick decision has to be made. The bonus of remaining conscious is that you will be ready to see and hold your baby as soon as it is delivered. However, some women prefer to be unconscious during surgery.

Emergency caesarians are performed when complications have developed during labour and delivery needs to be quick. Perhaps labour has failed to progress due to the baby being in an awkward position or the baby's head is too large to pass through the pelvis, or attempts to deliver the baby with forceps or vacuum extraction have failed.

A caesarian section can also be planned be advance, known as "elective", if labour is felt to be dangerous for the woman or baby. The baby may be lying in an awkward position, such as in the breech position, or the placenta may be lying over the cervix so preventing the baby's passage. Some women choose to have an elective caesarian section because they wish to avoid labour, or perhaps because their previous baby was born by emergency caesarian.

Because it involves major abdominal surgery, recovery after a caesarian section often takes longer than after vaginal delivery. A woman usually spends four to five days in hospital and is advised to avoid heavy lifting for several weeks (see also Physical Discomforts, p67).

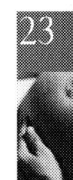

CAESARIAN RATE COMPARISONS
London   24%
(highest in UK)
Scandinavia   13%
USA   22%
Brazil   35%

The Rise in Caesarian Sections

Caesarians are widely regarded by obstetricians as more dangerous to maternal health than a vaginal birth (whereas about half the obstetricians in this country believe caesarians to be safer for the baby than a vaginal delivery). A concensus conference by the World Health Organisation in 1985 concluded that there were no additional health benefits associated with a caesarian section rate above 10–15%. Despite such attitudes, caesarian section delivery rates are climbing steadily in the UK. From under 3% in the 1950s, the rate had risen to 12% by 1990, and to 18% by 1997. According to the National Sentinel Caesarian Section Audit Report of 2001, the rate is now over 20%. In the report, the four main medical indications given for performing caesarian sections are failure to progress, foetal distress, breech presentation and repeat caesarian section.

Reasons for the rise are much debated and are likely to be due to a number of factors. In cases where, for example, the baby is in the breech position, obstetricians may prefer to carry out a caesarian section rather than to adopt other strategies such as turning the baby before labour begins.

Another factor accounting for the rise is that more women are choosing elective caesarians. The rate for these was up from 5% in 1981 to 8% in 1997/98. Reasons may include not wanting to go through labour and wanting to avoid difficulties that can occur after vaginal delivery such as incontinence, piles, or problems with an episiotomy healing. Others may have been traumatised by having a difficult labour with their first child, leading to an emergency caesarian, and prefer a planned caesarian second time around. The higher incidence of multiple pregnancies – often through fertility treatment – is also a factor.

Looking more closely at national figures, great significance has been drawn from the fact that caesarean section rates vary considerably between hospitals in different parts of the country. Some hospitals report a rate as low as 12%, while others report a 29% rate. *The Good Birth Guide*, published in 2001 by *The Sunday Times* in association with Dr Foster, an independent source of information about standards in UK healthcare, publishes figures for every maternity unit in the UK. From this, it can be seen that Southwest England has the highest rate of home births and the lowest rate of caesarians; the Northeast has the best levels of midwife staffing and a relatively low caesarian rate; the Southeast has some of the lowest levels of midwife staffing and the third highest rate of caesarians; the West Midlands has the highest rate of caesarians, but other forms of intervention are below the national average, including the lowest rate of epidurals.

Midwife shortages are likely to be part of the problem. Both the Royal College of Midwives and the National Childbirth Trust point out that the right kind of one-to-one support from a skilled midwife for every woman throughout labour would lead to a fall in rates for caesarians as well as for other interventions. The problem of midwife shortages is looked at in more detail below.

THE MIDWIFE CRISIS

Midwives have long been applauded for their dedication to their work and for the tremendous support they provide for women in labour, as well as during and after pregnancy. But in Britain, the service they offer is being seriously undermined by chronic shortfalls in NHS resources, and low morale. The result is, at present, a severe shortage of midwives both entering and staying in the profession, a situation that has been dubbed "the midwife crisis".

A survey undertaken by the Royal College of Midwives in July 2000 found that four out of five NHS maternity units have vacancies, with two out of three Heads of Midwifery describing staffing levels as "inadequate". The shortage is most acute in London where there is a 15% vacancy rate, and in the Southeast, where it is 7.5%, but there are also shortages in almost every other part of the country. Long-term vacancies (lasting at least four months) are rising in Scotland, the Northwest, the Southwest and Trent regions. Hence, midwives are having to cope with increasingly long hours and heavy workloads in a pressurised and stressful environment, usually on inadequate pay.

Inevitably, these problems are affecting how women experience childbirth and the quality of care that they receive. For instance, a woman may not have a midwife with her throughout labour because the midwife has to attend to other women; or she may be supported by a series of midwives she hasn't met before. Or perhaps she planned a home birth but finally gives birth in hospital because no midwife is available. Spontaneous labour and delivery – where the baby is delivered by a midwife – is also less likely, according to a study by the Royal College of Midwives, in a maternity unit with severe staffing problems. Staff shortages are therefore leading to increases in intervention rates and the medicalisation of maternity care, the survey concludes.

The support offered antenatally and postnatally is also affected by the shortage, with women more likely to receive care from large numbers of midwives or a midwife who they do not know. There may also be time pressures on appointments which can affect the quality of the discussion which takes place.

OTHER PROBLEMS IN MATERNITY SERVICES

In a survey conducted by the National Childbirth Trust in 1999, one in four women thought that health professionals had not always explained what was happening, or why certain things were being done, and did not take enough notice of their views and wishes. Bed shortages are another problem facing some NHS hospitals, so that some women have to be transferred to another hospital. Generally, women are staying in hospital for less time after birth than in previous decades. Where delivery is straightforward, the average stay tends to be about two days, but in certain areas, women are going home within a few hours. Whilst this may be welcomed by some, others may feel they would benefit from additional time in hospital. Surveys make it clear that women want maternity services that are woman-centred and responsive to individual needs.

LONG-TERM OUTLOOK

To ease the midwife crisis and to make services more woman-centred, the Government announced a series of measures in May 2001. These include better pay for midwives, incentives for returners to the profession, and the creation of

Interventions and the Midwife Crisis

more senior midwifery posts. Extra money is also to be made available to upgrade maternity units – both in terms of equipment and facilities, for instance more single rooms on maternity wards. Other goals have also been established, for example, every woman having access to a dedicated midwife when in established labour, and greater choices in childbirth – including home births – for all women. Antenatal and postnatal care should also be available from a known, trusted midwife.

There are also a number of people calling for more midwife-led units (see p14) to be made available. Skilled midwives can avoid the need for many interventions by a range of strategies, such as encouraging active birth principles to help a woman get through the pain without needing an epidural. Significance has been drawn from the fact that at the midwife-led Edgware Birth Centre in London, just 12% of women were transferred to hospital during labour, and even then, intervention rates were significantly lower than the national figures: 5% of women had an episiotomy, 11.4% had an epidural, and 3.9% were assisted with forceps or ventouse. Being in a more relaxed and sympathetic environment where you are supported by a midwife who can empathise with you and concentrate on your individual needs can make the experience of labour more positive. This contrasts with hospitals where there are sometimes set guidelines on the length of time a woman should continue in labour before an intervention takes place.

On the other hand, it is also worth remembering that women who go to midwife-led units are self-selecting because they are deemed to be "low risk". Many women are actually reassured by the presence of high-tech equipment, and prefer to give birth in hospital. Thus, broadening the availability of the range in services is the key.

Whether services become more woman-centred remains to be seen. But there are signs that the midwife crisis is receiving greater recognition than ever before, and that steps are being taken to improve the quality of care received by women and their babies at this crucial time in their lives.

Making the Most of Current Services

The editor of this book asked some mothers how they felt about maternity services in this country. Most had given birth in the local NHS hospital, and it appeared to be hit or miss as to whether they felt the effects of the midwife crisis and other problems. Annette had the most positive outloook. "From my experience and stories from friends and family, I think childbirth facilities in this country are pretty good. I personally received a fantastic amount of care from my NHS hospital and was always made aware of what was happening at every

---

MATERNITY PRACTICE ISSUES
For more information on the midwife crisis and other issues:

Association for Improvements in Maternity Services
01753 652781
www.aims.org.uk

Association of Radical Midwives
62 Greetby Hill
Ormskirk
Lancashire
L39 2DT
01695 572776
arm@radmid.
demon.co.uk

stage of my labour and birth." Jane S. and Melissa were also positive – both had been lucky enough to have several dedicated NHS midwives on the day.

Charlotte had chosen her hospital because it had a good reputation for neonatal care, was near to her home and had a Domino Scheme (see p15). "But in reality, the Domino Scheme wasn't working because of a shortage of midwives. The standard of postnatal care was appalling, particularly with respect to hygiene." Julia said that she didn't feel that she really had a choice – either about being in hospital or which hospital. "My impression of childbirth facilities in this country are that they seem adequate, but not brilliant. The staff are overburdened and only seem to focus on "problems" rather than providing support for women with "normal" pregnancies." Rhiann had suffered from the effects of the midwife shortage for her first birth, and hired an independent midwife for her second. "This was much better than my experience in hospital for our first child, in which I had a c-section in a room full of strangers, but we had to extend the mortgage to pay for her services."

If you are reading this while pregnant, then you might well wonder how the current shortfalls in maternity services might affect you. Indeed, it might be worth enquiring about any potential problems you might encounter, such as the likelihood of midwife availability for a home birth, or the statistical possibility of transfer from a low-tech to high-tech hospital in the event of complications. Having a labour companion will be all the more important if the midwife has to leave you alone for hours at a time. Ask other local mothers about their experiences. Jane S. was aware that there was a 50% transfer rate for first-time mothers from her cottage hospital to the high-tech ward at Exeter. Thus she was not too surprised or upset when advised to transfer during labour because her baby had started to show signs of distress. By contrast, Amy wasn't aware that there might not be a midwife available for her planned home birth in the London borough of Hackney, and she was desperately disappointed at having to go into hospital for her first birth. Events transpired to enable her to have her second child at home.

The issue of intervention rates and the promotion of midwifery are wrapped up with the politics of medicalised birth versus natural birth, which are explored more fully in the next section. To end this section on as positive a note as possible (having just painted a depressing picture of current maternity services), the editor would like to point out that at least at the time of writing there was no known compromise on safety due to the midwife shortages. Somehow or other, our country's understaffed maternity units are as safe to give birth in as those in other developed nations. It's just that you might feel like you are being herded on a conveyor belt in some of them…

Birth Politics

From what we hear and learn about birth from different sources – books, classes and other people – attitudes can often seem to be polarised between the medical establishment and natural birth movement. Here, **Kate Figes** looks at the way these attitudes developed and how they affect ordinary women.

ABOUT KATE FIGES
Kate Figes is a leading journalist and the author of Life After Birth: What Friends Won't Tell You About Motherhood (Penguin).

A Short History of Childbirth

The prospect of childbirth is usually daunting, particularly for women who are about to give birth for the first time. It isn't made any easier by the fact that women are faced with two polarised systems of managing labour which often seem to contradict one another. In one camp there is the NHS and the medical establishment, complete with foetal monitoring, pain relief and guaranteed intervention to save the lives of either mother or baby should it be necessary. In the opposite camp is the natural birth movement, which has been highly influential since the 1970s and successful at inculcating the view that much of this intervention is not only unnecessary, but also potentially harmful to the natural process of labour.

Between these two opposing stools fall countless ordinary women, who are ill-equipped to fight their corner against the mighty medical establishment because they are so vulnerable in labour. Most women are only certain that they want to do everything possible to protect the health of their baby as well as their perineum.

The history of childbirth relates that both arguments have right on their side. Little more than a hundred years ago, when labour was obstructed or prolonged, caesarean surgery was rarely successful, and countless babies were torn limb from limb in order to save the more important life of the mother. Maternal death from childbirth as well as severe postnatal health difficulties were common until the middle of the 20th century. Women died principally from illegal abortions and puerperal fever, although heamorrhage and toxaemia were also causes. Almost half of all the women who died in childbirth during the 19th and early 20th century, were struck down by sepsis in the days after delivering their child. Antibiotics and a clearer understanding of how infection spreads through open wounds, particularly in hospitals, led to a dramatic reduction in the death rate from puerperal fever, from 200 per 100,000 in 1935, to just 1 in 1960.

THE LONG MONTHS OF PREGNANCY

With such a high death rate prior to the medical advances of the mid-20th century onwards, childbirth was widely feared in a way that few of us can imagine today. Every woman would more than likely have known others who had died giving birth. Countless others were left with chronic health problems after labour such as lesions, and prolapsed wombs which were left untreated because healthcare had to be paid for and poor women inevitably put their needs last. There was no pain relief other than chloroform, which was expensive. Ordinary women just had to grin and bear it. Modern obstetric developments such as forceps, which do not rip the head off the baby, and epidurals, which allow the mother to stay awake while her baby is born by caesarean section, are definite advances for which we must be thankful.

But there are also ways in which the medical establishment has over-reacted to the risks of childbirth. Many of the deaths from childbed fever were caused by conditions within the new lying-in hospitals established during the 18th century, for doctors were unaware that they were transmitting infection from one woman to another often with their bare hands. With antibiotics, legalised abortion, less absolute poverty and healthier women, we are unlikely to return to the high risks of the past. For centuries women gave birth at home with midwives until they were persuaded and cajoled into hospitals towards the end of the 19th century. In hospitals doctors and consultants took control of the management of labour, and inevitably we have lost a great deal of midwifery expertise as a result.

A PERSPECTIVE ON SAFETY
It is women in the developing world who now suffer 99% of maternal deaths. They are dying needlessly at a rate of 600,000 per year for many of the same reasons that European women died up until the 1930s – infection, haemorrhage, abortion and toxaemia.

The natural birth movement has helped in some ways to haul the medical establishment back into some sort of reasonable centre ground. The books of Grantly-Dick Read in the 1930s were the first to express concern over the way women were controlled through labour. The works of Lamaze and then Sheila Kitzinger in the 1960s and 1970s took the baton still further. Through extensive research and lobbying, these and other influential figures managed to persuade many doctors that women do not need to be shaved or have routine enemas before labour, that lying on their backs is not necessarily the most comfortable, logical or successful way to deliver a baby and that episiotomies need to be reserved for emergencies. Tears may be more difficult to sew, but episiotomies cut deeper into the muscle tissue, tend to be more painful and take longer to heal. Hospital may be the most convenient and cheapest way for the state to deliver babies, but the high-tech atmosphere can frighten women unduly, slowing down the first stage of labour. The caesarean rate may not

Caesarian in the late Middle Ages (below).

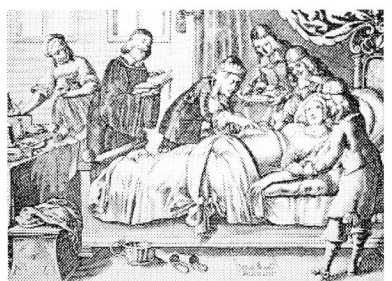

be as high in the UK as it is in the US, where doctors principally fear litigation. But it is far too high and rising because of the factory farming method of managing labour, where women are routinely hooked onto monitors and drips, have their labours speeded up and lack proper one-to-one midwifery care.

Expectations of Birth

While the natural birth movement has been partially successful in moderating the exuberance of male obstetricians and highlighting the lamentable downgrading of midwives, it has also heaped new pressures and expectations on women. The emphasis on the natural aspects of pregnancy and childbirth diminishes the great discomfort that so many women feel during pregnancy. They know that pregnancy is not an illness, but nevertheless feel ill much of the time. The emphasis on avoiding pain relief because drugs can inhibit labour and pass through the lining of the womb to the baby places countless women in an intolerable self-sacrificial position. Childbirth is usually the most painful experience on God's Earth, but the baby has to come first.

Women who have never given birth before imagine that they will be able to control the intensity of that pain through yogic breathing alone. Then when the textbook theory turns into reality, breathing technique often evaporates and women beg for pain relief. If they develop complications and need forceps or end up having a caesarean, all too often women feel as if they have failed. They feel inadequate as mothers before they have even begun. They feel disappointed at their performance, at their weakness in the face of drugs as well as shock at the stark reality of labour.

Now that death in childbirth is less likely than dying in a road accident, we seem to have replaced the fears that women lived with just a hundred years ago with fear of pain and an episiotomy. The ideology of natural birth tends to create presumptions in women that there is a right and a wrong way to give birth, that it can be prepared for like some sort of exam and that women can and must control and actively manage the progress of their labour.

What the ideology tends to overlook is the fact that labour is often unpredictable. While there are usually three defined stages to childbirth, there is no way of knowing how those stages will progress, how long a woman will spend in each or how she will react to them. Doctors and midwives know that no two labours are ever the same even in the same woman, and that complications can rarely be predicted. That's why they tend to fall so hard on the side of caution. And while the theory of managing your labour, saying what you want and don't want and remaining in control is all very well, often what women discover is that labour controls them. Giving birth means giving in to your body, to the great waves of contractions and often trying to stay in control is counterproductive. For centuries women in labour have needed caring midwives constantly at their side to explain and soothe simply because they are so vulnerable and out of control at this time. To expect otherwise is simply unreasonable.

The point of childbirth is to have a baby and become a mother. The process itself is in most women's eyes temporary and best forgotten. The trouble with much of the ideology of natural birth is that the emphasis is on labour itself, with teachers who are fascinated by the birth process, and not on the aftermath, which can be devastating, physically and emotionally. Often feelings of failure in childbirth contribute to postnatal unhappiness, a factor which would have been unheard of in the past. Postnatal support is lamentable in the UK. Women are routinely dismissed at six weeks even though ill health lingers on and visits from midwives and health visitors cease. Women need the support of other new mothers desperately at this time and the friendships formed at antenatal classes can be invaluable. But if new mothers feel as if they have failed because they have had a caesarean, if they feel inadequate and depressed because they cannot cope, they are unlikely to return to these groups of friends and feel even more isolated.

With such polarised views on the management of labour, the women who are most vulnerable and most in need of support often feel caught in between, which is a great shame. They want to have as easy a time as possible in labour, but they also want to do their best for their baby. They have no choice but to subscribe to the state system of antenatal care and childbirth, which they have good reason to fear, and yet the only alternative available seems equally extreme.

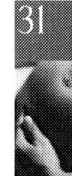

What pregnant women need ideally is the best of both worlds, a system that treats each woman individually and supports her adequately through a unique and extraordinary experience that is natural but can be dangerous. In an ideal world, medical intervention would be kept to a minimum and women would be free from guilt about the individual choices they make with pain relief or even elective caesarean. Until the day when these two warring extremes meet in the middle, individual women have little choice but to pick their way through a minefield and remember some basic truths: childbirth rarely matches the idyll of natural birth ethos and is usually far more painful than women imagine it will be; childbirth has always been difficult for human beings because we give birth to young with such large heads, but it is far safer now in the Western world than it has ever been. Childbirth is a profound rite of passage for women and needs to be welcomed and cherished as such. No woman emerges from it unchanged or unscarred in some way. Our bodies change and so do our priorities as they have done for millions and millions of women before.

Views on Birth Politics

The editor asked various people for their views on the polarisation between medical and natural birth. Statements from **Sheila Kitzinger**, independent midwife **Andrea Dombrowe** and President of the Royal College of Obstetricians and Gynaecologists, **William Dunlop**, are included, followed by views from mothers themselves.

Sheila Kitzinger

"Natural childbirth" is a much misused term. In fact, I have never used it, because it is open to so much misunderstanding. Must you squat in the woods with the wild things? Are you less of a woman if you decide you require obstetric help? If you have a caesarean, does it mean you have "failed"?

"Natural childbirth" doesn't mean much, either. All birth in human beings is a matter of culture. As a social anthropologist, I study different patterns of birth across the globe. Many of them support physiological, or normal, birth. Our own medicalised and technocratic culture of birth is impressive when there is pathology, but fails to support normal, physiological processes. The result is that women today may experience birth as a kind of rape. Babies are "saved" by caesarean sections, and their mothers are chopped up and sewn together again. Women are not only abused, but when they are distressed after childbirth are urged to be grateful that they have a live, healthy baby and to put the birth behind them and get on with their lives. Post-traumatic stress affects not only new mothers, but their relationships with their partners and babies, and may continue for months – even years.

When a labour is going well and a woman is able to be in tune with the rhythms of her body, without intrusion, the waves of contractions are exhilarating, and she responds to them spontaneously with breathing, relaxation and movement. She would no more want someone to deaden the intense sensations with drugs, or to take over the birth of her baby, than she would want someone to anaesthetise or assist her when she was making love. Indeed, the same hormones flood into her bloodstream and stimulate her uterus that pour through her when she is sexually aroused. Yes, there is pain. But when she is overwhelmed with excitement and with wonder at the creative power of her body it becomes positive pain – pain with a purpose.

There are great skills, involving art and science, in supporting normal childbirth. These are midwifery skills. They entail sensitive awareness and an understanding of how women's bodies work. They also demand an understanding of research evidence, so that caregivers are aware of the side-effects for the mother and her baby of interventions like confining labouring women to bed, electronically monitoring the foetal heartbeat, offering drugs for pain relief in the absence of strong emotional support, telling women to push and hold their breath, and episiotomy.

The politics of birth care are often discussed in terms of a spurious "post-feminism" and a woman's right to choose whatever kind of birth she wants. But they also need to be explored in terms of coercion, persuasion and obstetric "birth speak", in terms of our fear and problems of coping with it. It is impossible that medicine should provide an answer to all our woes, all our suffering, and through the administration of drugs and quick resort to surgery, leave our lives free of stress, striving and challenge.

Bringing new life into the world should never be reduced to being equivalent to the removal of a decayed molar or a septic appendix. However complicated the birth, everyone involved should work in harmony to make it a joyful and triumphant experience. The birth of each child is for the mother, her partner and the whole family a life transition of deep and lasting significance."

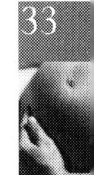

ABOUT SHEILA KITZINGER
The birth research and campaigns of Sheila Kitzinger are summarised on pp17–18.

ANDREA DOMBROWE

"We have to bring normality back into birth! It is not a disease or a problem to be managed, but is and can be a normal, beautiful and empowering event, encompassing the whole family. The fear of litigation and hospital policies which are not always research-based often treat birthing women like machines, who have to complete their "programme" within a timescale; if not, their labour is often actively managed. No wonder some hospitals have a caesarean section rate of 28%. Women need to feel secure, know their midwife and build their confidence in themselves and their ability to birth gently. But where are the midwives, and not obstetric nurses, to give them this confidence? Midwives need to stand up together as the autonomous practitioners they are, for all women!"

WILLIAM DUNLOP

"The idea of polarisation between the medical profession and the natural birth movement is outdated and misleading. It perpetuates the thinking of a decade ago. It is essential that those who have a professional involvement in serving women and children during pregnancy and childbirth accept women's right to choose and support them in the decisions that they make. Women's

Views on Birth Politics

representatives are now working closely with midwives and obstetricians to produce a National Service Framework for maternity services for the next decade. This is a unique opportunity to improve the care of mothers and babies in the United Kingdom."

Mothers' Views on Birth Politics

As is often the case when an amorphous body of ideas gains influence and gets called a "movement", the natural birth movement means different things to different people. Out of the 50, or so, women interviewed for this book, five said they had never heard of a natural birth movement or active birth principles. Others had their own opinions on what they thought the politics were all about, and some felt caught in the middle – let down by both the medical establishment and what they perceived to be the ideology of "natural birth".

Deborah, Amy and Melissa were among those who were very positive about the natural birth movement and felt that following active birth principles helped immensely. "I am hugely grateful to the movement for turning the tide on routinely medicalised birth," writes Deborah. "I did midwife-led classes before having my first child and found them less helpful than talking to relatives and friends who are mothers, and reading, especially Sheila Kitzinger's *Pregnancy and Childbirth*, which I loved. My first birth was "old-fashioned", with a consultant obstetrician "in charge" and midwives very subservient. When I was expecting my second child I read a lot about natural birth, bolstered by yoga classes. My second birth in a low-tech maternity unit was very, very positive as a result."

Melissa's story of her water birth is on p49. Her mother and sisters had also had good childbirth experiences, and she had been relieved to find herself in the care of no fewer than five midwives on the day – not an obstetrician in sight during either labour or delivery. "I consider myself lucky in so many ways," she says, "because not only have I perhaps inherited a body that gives birth with relative ease, but fate also brought me an available birthing pool and supportive midwives on the day. Stories from friends show that many are not so lucky."

Julia said she likes the mother and baby centred approach of the natural birth movement, but is also a bit critical. "The technological and medical approach needed to be challenged. However, I feel the whole movement is very white and middle class and does not address the needs of women with low income, no partner or a poor education, who cannot access books and expensive courses." Julia's birth was fairly straightforward, and she resisted the midwife's suggestion to artificially break her waters. Her story is on p38.

THE POLITICS OF BIRTH PLANS
The trend for writing a birth plan, in which you set out your preferences on medical interventions and other issues, is related to birth politics. The plan shows your birth support team how you feel about the use of pain relief, induction etc.

The editor's view is that birth plans are largely unnecessary. It is good to learn about the pros and cons of interventions in advance, but dialogue with your midwives will surely be worth more than a written statement. Going into hospital with a written plan can make your preferences seem absolute and create conflict on the day. (See also p71).

Charlotte was also ambivalent. She had written a birth plan saying that she wanted as natural a birth as possible, but her labour turned out to be long and excruciating, culminating in a forceps delivery (see p50). When asked what she thought about the natural birth movement, she said, "As far as I am aware, the movement consists of a philosophy that labour should involve as little medical intervention as possible. I presume it advocates the use of natural pain relief (such as TENS, breathing techniques, massage, water) and also advocates home birth. My opinion is that all this is great for straightforward labours, but pain-killing drugs do have a valuable role to play, if (and it's a big if) they are administered with care. Home births are a great idea if you happen to live near a hospital."

Ruth was forthright in her criticism of the ideology of natural birth. "I was always sceptical of the view that birth should be attempted or be desirable with the minimum of drugs and intervention, the more so after my personal experience of a labour full of complications, culminating in an emergency caesarian. This perhaps stems from my experience in developing countries as a journalist. "Natural birth" in rural Cambodia, for example, means pain, trauma and high risk for mother and child. I find it incomprehensible that some women here aspire to, and are encouraged towards, a birth where "intervention" or drugs means "failure". Medical procedures are not an optional extra, but an essential support without which millions of women worldwide suffer indescribable pain and death. Those who preach against medical help are romanticising childbirth." See Ruth's birth story on p40.

Alice was one of those women who were critical of both the medical establishment and the idea of having a natural birth without intervention. "In some ways I believe that the natural birth movement is performing a very valuable role, as childbirth should not automatically be viewed as a medical procedure. However, I think that a little more realism would be apt with regard to the ability of women in their mid-30s (quite a common age for middle-class British women with whom the movement is most closely associated), to give birth "naturally". I am very fit and healthy, yet becoming a mother at nearly 33, my body was just not up to the job of giving birth to a large baby. At least that's my take on it. Because one of my disappointments at the whole birth experience is the lack of medical follow-up, particularly for women who intend to have more children. I have absolutely no idea why I ended up having a caesarian, when I'd intended to have a drug-free water birth. Should I just assume that I should elect for a c-section for my next baby? Why do I have to rely on my own instincts and not on medical care for this?" Her story is on p41.

LOW AND POSITIVE EXPECTATIONS
Hopefully in the future, midwifery pressures will ease, and birth practice will become more geared to the individual needs of women.

Besides this, the editor's view is that it's actually good to build up an expectation that birth will be arduous, whether intervention is used or not – your expectations then can't be dashed so easily. Include a scenario of caesarian in your dreams about birth.

Also bear in mind that labour is usually a matter of hours – a few days at the most. Birth may be a huge event in itself, but it is also a relatively short moment that will pale next to the tremendous time to follow.

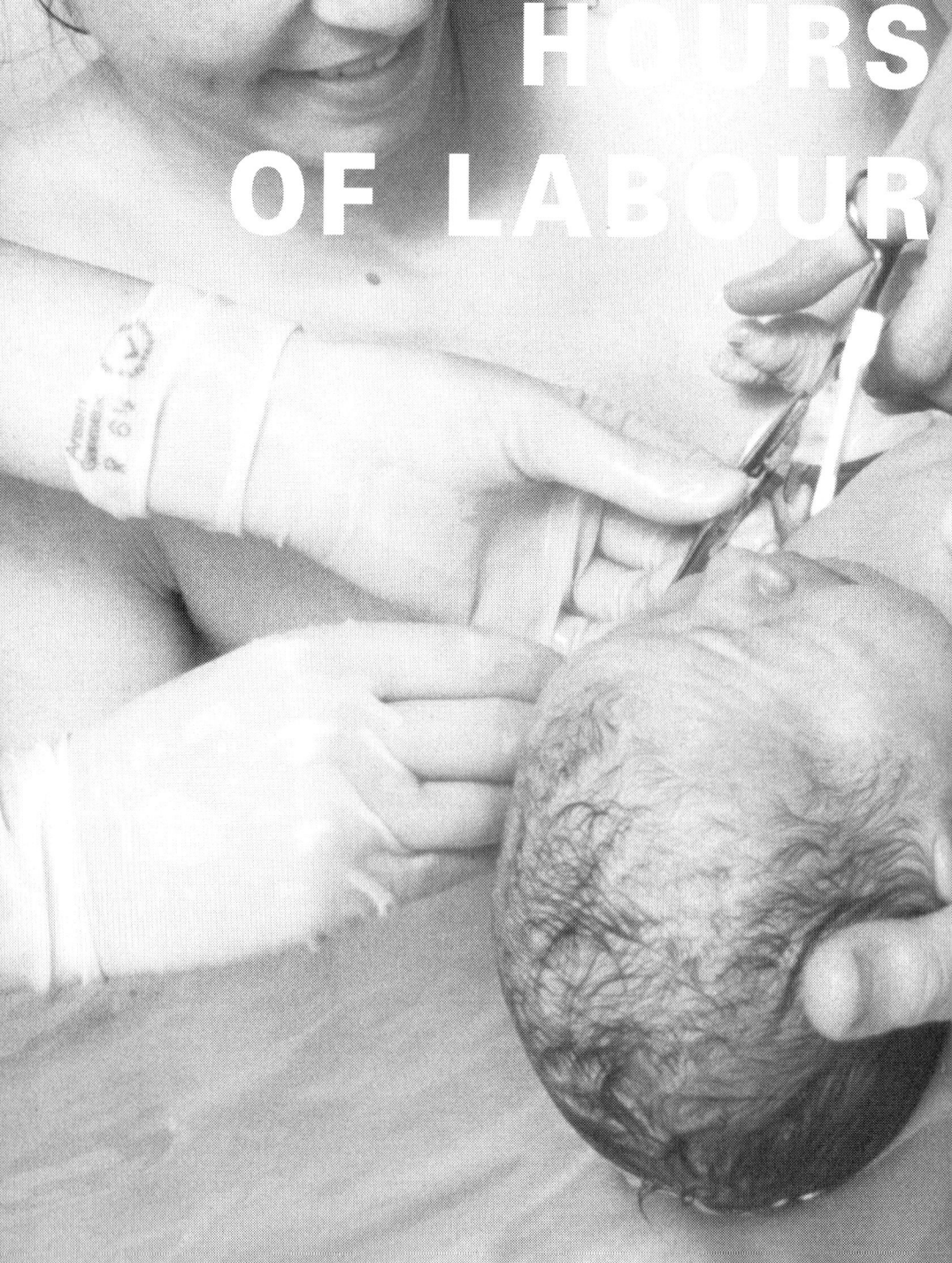

THE HOURS OF LABOUR

37

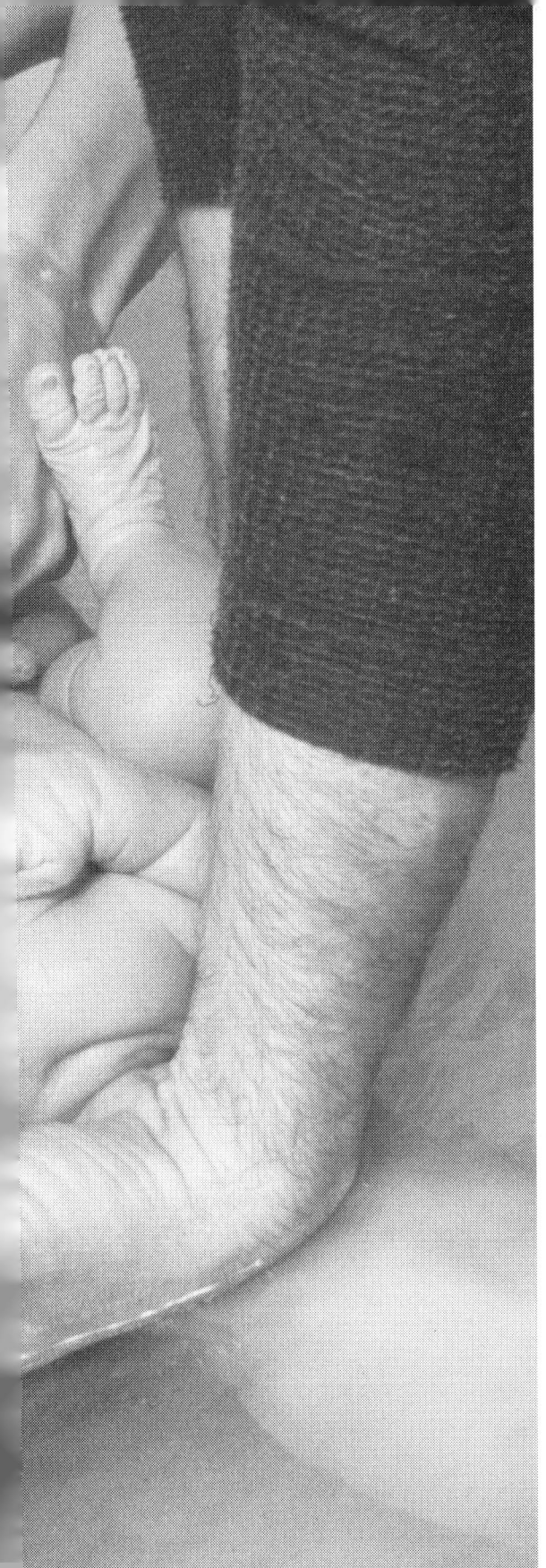

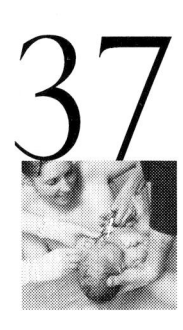

Contents

38 Real Birth Stories

52 A Closer Look at Labour Pain

Real Birth Stories

There may be lots of information about the process of birth and pain relief, but the real enlightenment comes from mothers. Some elements of the selected birth stories here are common to the experiences of labouring women everywhere; other parts are specific to the experience of childbirth in modern Britain.

Birth as a Sequence of Events

The editor invited some women who had recently become mothers to tell their birth stories, from the first signs of labour to delivery. The selection of stories was made to be representative of certain types of delivery and intervention: varying lengths of labour, the use of different forms of pain relief, normal vaginal delivery, forceps and ventouse, emergency and elective caesarian, and one water birth. They are all first births. Such is the high drama of birth that even a small selection of stories, a couple of which are harrowing, is almost exhausting to read. A closer look at the experience of pain in labour is on pp52–57.

Julia's Story
On the expected date

"From early pregnancy I was convinced that my baby was going to be born on the fifth of August, three days late by official dating, her due date by my counting. On the eve of this date I sat down to dinner with my partner, David, poured myself a glass of wine, something I hadn't done for nine months, and commented that this would be our last meal on our own.

I went to bed, slept reasonably well and woke up feeling fine. However, by mid-morning a slight backache had appeared. By lunchtime there were contractions, sometimes a few minutes apart, sometimes 20 minutes. I was sitting in the bath full to the brim with warm water, still feeling calm, and decided to call the hospital. Whilst speaking on the phone I had a huge contraction and nearly dropped the handset in the bath. The midwife seemed sceptical of my view that I was now in established labour, but suggested I go in for a check.

We arrived at the hospital at 6.30pm and I was delighted to discover that I was already 5cm dilated. The midwife said she could feel the waters bulging out and asked if I wanted her to break them. Immediately I had to think – somehow logic took over – I've got far this already, so I don't need intervention, therefore don't break them. (The waters later broke naturally just as my baby was born, and it pleases me to think that this would have cushioned her head during birth.)

I decided to use gas and air and quickly got into a rhythm of breathing: I used the gas and air as each contraction peaked, then switched to the breathing learnt in antenatal yoga as it lessened and stopped. David helped by rubbing my back and manoeuvring me to a big cushion, which I slumped over to rest between each contraction.

At 9cm dilation I got the most overwhelming urge to push, while the midwives were changing shifts. I felt upset that the midwife I had been familiar with for months was leaving, and I was to give birth with a stranger. Soon afterwards, I was allowed to go ahead and push. This was a relief, but it was also frenzied, like I was acting on some uncontrollable animal instinct.

After a while I asked if the baby was making much progress. "Look", said David, and in our hand mirror I saw this tiny head of dark damp hair. I carried on pushing, still sucking on my gas and air pump, which had become my new best friend. Everything had been going so well up to this point, when the baby became stuck. The midwife and David looked at my tight skin around the baby's head: the midwife suggested an episotomy. I couldn't really think at all. Somehow we decided that I should move onto all fours, and as I started to move I had a massive contraction – it was too late, the baby was coming and I had to have the episiotomy. But I didn't mind being cut at that point, I felt that it time for her to be born. Then I pushed some more and out she came."

Baby Caitlin was born after about seven hours of labour. More of Julia's stories are on pp27, 34, 53, 56, 57 and 61.

ANNETTE'S STORY
Induction after the waters break

"My waters broke the night before my due date. Contractions were mild, but Tony and I went to the maternity unit for a check anyway. There was meconium in the waters, so a monitor was attached to keep tags on the baby's heart rate. Tony went back home while I was taken up to a ward overnight, with the monitor on constantly. I was told that I would be induced in the morning – to get the contractions going rather than risk infection because the waters had already broken. I didn't sleep much and was taken down at 8.30am to my delivery room.

Tony came back to the hospital, and they set up the drip to induce me. My midwife (a fantastic woman – extremely kind and caring) said that if I had an open mind about pain relief then she would advise an epidural because induction would make the contractions extremely intense and painful. I was

Annette with baby Annie

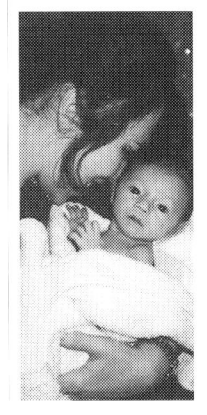

happy to go along with this, but in the meantime the doctor came in and gave me an internal and had to break my waters further, which was agony. It took two attempts for the anaesthetist to get the epidural in – more pain – however once it kicked in it really was worth having.

The scariest time during the whole labour was about an hour after I had been checked at 3cm dilation – the baby's heart rate suddenly dropped. Everyone was rushing round and the doctor came back in. Another check showed that I was fully dilated (much quicker than expected), and so the pushing began. About another hour later, and with the help of the ventouse, Annie was born."

Annette's labour was about two hours from the start of induction. See also her stories on pp26, 55, 61, 66, 70, 89, 121, 136, 147 and 205.

Ruth's Story
Multiple complications

"The first sign of labour was 12 hours of slow bleeding. Hence my arrival at hospital earlier than I might otherwise have done. I was having contractions but they were not too painful or frequent. What pushed the birth along was the monitor of the baby – showing signs of distress after some hours. So I had my waters broken (not disagreeable, despite my fears) and then I was induced.

Contractions were intense and I tried pethidine, but it didn't kill the pain. An epidural was offered, and it was total bliss. I was able to sleep after 24 hours of wakefulness and ready to push when I'd opened up enough. But nothing happened, even after one-and-a-half hours of full-power pushing. And so, a decision was made to go to surgery, either for forceps or emergency caesarian. I was hugely relieved to hear they would perform a caesarian because I had a powerful sense that I could not push this baby out.

The c-section was a strange episode – totally painless, but macabre. I felt powerful rummaging, as though someone had lost something in a sock drawer. It went on and on, punctuated by the odd spot of blood which leapt over the curtain, onto my specs at one point. The baby was so stuck in my pelvis that the female doctor was not strong enough to pull her out, and needed assistance from her male colleague. And then they held up this scowling, dark-haired baby girl and I smiled. It then took another 30 minutes of desperate rummaging. I later discovered that they pulled my uterus out of my abdomen in order to locate a bleed which cost 2 litres of blood. The worst part was the uncontrollable shivering, so strong I felt I might fall off the operating table, and a feeling of desperate cold. But I didn't care – there was a healthy baby girl!"

Rosa was born after a day and a half. Ruth's stories about the early months are on pp19, 35, 56, 57, 61, 64, 67, 68, 72, 88, 120, 203 and 204.

JUSTINE'S STORY
On-off contractions over three days

"My labour started with three contractions 30 minutes apart. This was exciting, but nothing happened for the rest of the day until evening. The pain was not too intense, even exhilirating, and the time between contractions was very loving with Mark, my partner. But then the contractions stopped again until the next morning, when they came every 10 minutes or so. After 24 hours of this we went to the hospital to find that I was only half a centimetre dilated, and learning this made me depressed and weepy. I was told I had a back labour and was advised to stay at home as long as possible and come in when I wanted pain relief. Eating and reading between contractions took me through another 24 hours, but then exhaustion (no sleep for three days and nights) and increasing pain prompted us to go back to the hospital.

My sister was there throughout helping me and my partner. I wanted a water birth, and as the bath was filling my waters broke (a wonderful feeling). Unfortunately there was meconium in my waters, so from that moment the baby was monitored. I felt a certain amount of movement from the baby, but the foetal heartbeat became irregular. The hospital staff said they needed to augment my contractions and suggested an epidural. I readily agreed to an epidural, as the only relief had been baths and yoga breathing through several days of debilitating pain.

The next five hours were scary, with the baby in distress at various points, and caesarian often mentioned. Suddenly I was fully dilated. We let the epidural wear off, then I felt a movement in my birth canal. Midwives checked; I pushed – 12 minutes later a wide awake baby girl was born!

I had massaged my perineum with baby oil every day from six months, and had strong pelvic floor muscles, so didn't tear. I enjoyed pushing and delivery, but probably because I had been longing to for several days! Three sets of midwives had helped, all lovely, and Ella fed from me in the delivery suite."

Justine's labour was three days long. For more of her stories, see pp19, 60, 65, 67, 70, 120, 136, 192, 205, 208, 220 and 233.

ALICE'S STORY
Four days of exhausting "twinges"

"I expected to miss my due date which was a Thursday and kept telling people that I thought it would be on the Sunday afterwards. In fact, I had my first twinge on the Saturday night. Stomach cramps began and continued for the next 12 hours. They were no worse than period pain, but they meant that I had my first bad night's sleep of many. For the rest of Sunday I had quite regular contractions. I began using a TENS machine that I'd hired and overall the contractions were not unbearable. My partner, Richard, was timing the length and regularity of the contractions and at around midnight on Sunday we thought that they were regular enough that we should go into the birth centre (a low-tech, midwife-led centre).

The midwife told me that I had not even begun to dilate, and that I was just having "twinges", so should go home until I was really in labour. I felt really humiliated by this, as I'd been having regular contractions for around eight hours and even though the pain was not particularly intense, it seemed unbelievable that these were just twinges and not real labour. On Monday I carried on having contractions and felt nauseous. My community midwife suggested Lucozade, but after one sip of it, I was so violently sick that I gave myself a nosebleed. This was one of the real low points of the labour.

On Tuesday morning, a hospital examination showed that I was now 3–4cm dilated – proper labour. I was SO happy about that, as I'd felt really lost not knowing whether I was making any progress at all. So we went back to the birth centre, where midwives made regular checks. Once my contractions had intensified I was allowed to use the pool and also encouraged to get out and walk up and down the corridor every few hours to keep things going.

Around midnight on Tuesday I was examined again, but discovered that I had made virtually no progress at all since the morning. The midwife recommended that I be transferred to the nearest hospital and induced to speed things up. As I had been in labour for so long and was very tired – missing my third night's sleep and still unable to eat anything – I agreed and gave up my goal of having a natural water birth. I'd never been in an ambulance before, but everything was strange at that point, so it was just another new experience. I had decided that I could not cope with the pain of induction without more pain relief, so I had an epidural. It was administered, rather clumsily, by an extremely rude doctor, with whom I practically had an argument, despite my condition!

So I was in a labour room, in a hospital gown, strapped to a monitor with no sensation any more. I had some sleep then, at last. Richard was sitting in a chair in the room and I can't imagine to this day how he was feeling at the time. I think it was in the hospital that everything became truly shocking for him to watch as it was much more "medical" and less natural than in the birth centre.

At around 6am on Wednesday morning, the midwife examined me again and thought that I was now fully dilated and ready to start pushing when the epidural wore off a bit. She broke my waters with a crochet hook or something which sounds horrible, but I didn't really feel a thing. During all of this, the monitor had shown that the baby was somehow fine.

I pushed for around 45 minutes and absolutely hated it. It was the worst bit of labour. I also felt really negative and defeatist about the whole thing. Somehow I just knew that it wasn't working. I also couldn't stand the fact that it was like doing a poo – with lots of people, including my partner, watching. I made him stand towards my head so he couldn't really see what was going on down there.

I was told to stop pushing, which was hard as the pain was quite bad then and it was difficult not to push. Then a group of people suddenly came into the room, led by a woman in a summer suit with a handbag, looking like a visiting MP or something. She asked if she could put some questions to me and, totally misunderstanding the situation, I told her that "it wasn't really the right time for that". She was actually the consultant doctor, who was just coming onto her shift, had seen my records and thought that I needed immediate attention. She examined me internally and pronounced that the baby was posterior (facing backwards) and appeared to have got stuck. So she said I should have a caesarian.

I immediately agreed to the caesarian. So many of my friends have had them, that I just felt like I was joining their club. Also I just wanted labour to be over. It had been going on for so long – three days – and I somehow knew that I wasn't going to get the baby out myself. So I was wheeled into the operating theatre where a very chatty and jolly team of doctors had just begun their shift. Richard and I were having quite a nice time talking to the anaesthetist who had topped up my epidural, so that I was totally numb below the armpits. (I think I was their first operation of the day, and midwives have since commented on how neat my scar is!)

Before I even knew that they'd opened me up, we heard a baby's cry and realised that the child had been born. I hadn't felt a thing. They took the baby away before they showed it to us and so it was only after a few minutes when we saw it and found out that it was a boy – an amazing moment that I can still remember quite clearly."

Alice's four-day labour and caesarian left trauma in its wake. Her anecdotes are on pp35, 65, 68, 71, 87, 121, 213 and 221.

Jane's Story
Straightforward first stage, then difficulty with the second

"My labour started with a show at 7.30'ish in the morning and period-like discomfort. By lunchtime the twinges had grown into occasional contractions. By 5pm contractions were coming once every ten minutes or so. A friend had popped round for a cup of tea and I remember having to break off the conversation while I did my deep breathing. That evening I spent a lot of time deep breathing and making low moaning sounds (as practised in the yoga class) while crouching on all fours, leaning over the back of the sofa or slumped over a beanbag. I also found lying in a warm bath really helpful. At around 8pm the contractions had got a lot stronger and were coming every five minutes so I phoned the hospital and we were told to come in.

After a quick but uncomfortable journey (speed bumps during labour aren't recommended) I was admitted but we had to wait a while – maybe an hour – before I could be examined. When the midwife did examine me I was 6cm dilated. Tim and I were both amazed and elated. The contractions were unbelievably painful but I felt I was managing. Around this time I also started using gas and air, which felt heavenly. The birthing pool became available, and I remember sitting in this wonderful, warm bath feeling ridiculously happy. The atmosphere seemed very informal and intimate. I recall chatting away to Tim and the two midwives between contractions.

At 9cm dilation, the midwife said she reckoned the baby would be born within an hour or so. Things began to go less smoothly during the second stage. I spent ages trying to master the pushing technique but nothing was happening. I didn't experience any desire to push and was making no progress. Eventually I had to leave the birthing pool and go to the maternity suite so the baby could be monitored.

More time passed and when the registrars started hovering I knew that an intervention was on the cards. Things then start to get hazy. We had to wait around one-and-a-half hours for a delivery suite to become available. I was then moved to a high-tech suite complete with stirrups and hooked up to a drip to strengthen my weakening contractions. Then they took away the gas and air, which made me feel scared but also angry – by then it was my essential companion. I wanted to keep on pushing for a few more minutes but they said that the baby's heartbeat was getting weaker so they needed to intervene – this was two hours after hitting second stage.

The final few minutes were the most painful of all but passed by in what seemed like a flash. I was given a local anaesthetic and episiotomy and then they fitted a ventouse to the baby's head. But the only one available was too small and kept slipping off – his head was quite large. So the ventouse had to be removed, and the doctor declared she was going to try forceps instead. This felt as if all my insides were being yanked out, and I remember yelling in agony. Then this warm slippery creature was put onto my tummy and I burst into tears – sheer relief that labour was over and I had my baby at last."

Baby Angus was born about 24 hours after the show.

The Hours of Labour

Rosalyn's Story
High blood pressure two weeks early

"I was 38 weeks pregnant when my blood pressure suddenly rose. The senior obstetrician wanted to kick-start labour right away, with a membrance sweep. This consisted of her expertly pushing the bag of waters off the cervix with her finger, without breaking the waters. I was astonished when she said that I was already about 2cm dilated and she had touched the baby's head through the cervix. She predicted that labour would start within 48 hours.

As Mike, my partner, drove us home I started to feel period-like cramps, but I hoped that nothing more would happen that evening – until the previous day I had still assumed that there was at least two weeks to go, and had been working. Both of us needed a few hours, at least, to adjust to the idea that birth was imminent. We were lucky in this respect and even had a decent night's sleep.

I woke up at 7.30 the next morning, and as soon as I started moving little contractions began. They were lasting for about 10 seconds and coming every two to three minutes. This was surprising, as I had expected labour to start with contractions coming every half hour then pulling closer together. However, I could still walk and talk during these contractions, so I assumed they weren't the "real thing". After a few hours of this, we went for a walk and I felt really, incredibly calm. In the afternoon, I suggested to Mike that he go to buy the wood we needed to do a repair. The contractions were still coming every few minutes and still mild but I was becoming a bit irritated and wondering if this stage was going to continue for several days, which would be exhausting. While Mike was out I decided to drink some raspberry-leaf tea – even though I was skeptical that it would have much effect at "toning my uterus". My antenatal teacher had also recommended taking a bath to see if contractions either subsided or intensified. Within minutes contractions intensified to about 20 seconds each (I'm still too much of a skeptic to link it definitely to the tea). I splished in the bath for a bit then phoned Mike as I was alarmed at the change in gear. He returned just as I had got out of the bath and was gasping and swearing on the bed. I wanted to be in hospital: this definitely had to be the real thing.

I was relieved to get to the hospital, but took an instant dislike to the midwife assigned: she spent ages writing copious notes and barely saying a word to either of us. Because of my high blood pressure I had to be continuously monitored and would not be allowed to use the pool. Over the next couple of hours, as the contractions intensified

Rosalyn with baby Minna, six hours after forceps delivery

further, a terrible and constant backache appeared, which turned the miserable situation into a total nightmare. I hated being tethered to the monitors, and the gas and air did nothing to ease the pain. I was convinced that the canister must be empty, or if it was working, then it was merely serving to make me paranoid. People came in and out the room: I don't remember much of what was said. I started to believe that these were my last hours on Earth, just as giving birth to my father had been his mother's last hours.

There was a change in nursing shift, and my midwife's parting gesture was to tell me not to worry, that I was having very powerful contractions and that I would likely give birth before 2am. She meant this kindly, I know, and at least there was official acknowledgement that this was full-on labour, the worst of it. But 2am was seven hours away, and I knew that I could not possibly bear this level of pain for that amount of time. I asked pitifully for an epidural.

The new midwives were much kinder. I babbled to one that my father's mother had died in this process, and she said "poor thing" and stroked my legs, a strangely simple gesture that did bolster my feelings a bit. Various things were strapped to my back, but we had to wait for confirmation of some blood test before I was allowed the epidural. This took two hours, with me writhing around, groaning and trying to breathe.

At last the epidural arrived. The agonies driving through my body started to become numb. Within minutes the contrast was incredible, and I soon perked up emotionally and physically. Mike settled to read the paper while I dozed on and off through the night, clutching some Shinto charms for a safe childbirth. My contractions slowed – an effect of the epidural – so I was given a drip to artificially speed them up again. At one stage, the epidural was wearing off but no-one came to see us for hours. I was in deep fear of returning to the previous state of pain, and there was animal-like shrieking from other rooms – three women were giving birth at this time, so no staff were available. An extra dose of the epidural was given after this, and I managed to snooze a bit more.

By about 5.30am, I became aware of a pressure against my bottom and of the baby's feet pressing up into my diaphragm, which made me vomit. The midwife said that the baby was ready to be born, so I started pushing, though I couldn't really feel where I was pushing. I think the midwife was surprised that I managed to push the baby maybe halfway down despite the strength of the epidural. However, after an hour of pushing, the baby was still only halfway down and showing signs of distress.

Forceps were tentatively mentioned, and I immediately agreed, as I wanted this labour over and done with. This procedure was not nearly so horrible as I had previously imagined. I had shut my eyes and opened them again to find half a dozen total strangers in the room. An enormous, blood-covered creature was placed on my belly, and I gasped with emotion. Then it was carried over to the resuscitation table and started crying. After being cleaned and swaddled, an exquisitely beautiful baby girl was put in my arms…"

Baby Minna was born after exactly 24 hours of contractions. Rosalyn is the editor of Baby and You. More personal stories can be found in each chapter.

Claudia's Story
Relatively short but very intense labour

"I had a show three days before my due date. There were no contractions, but my boyfriend and I decided to go to the hospital for a checkup because I wasn't sure if my waters had also broken – a bit of clear fluid had been coming out for some time. The hospital monitor showed zero contractions in 20 minutes, so we were sent home. Another check the following day showed that there were still no contractions. My due date came and went, and the following day was also an anti-climax. The next morning seemed like it was going to be the same boring kind of day of waiting. Then at 10am I started having period pain in my belly. Fred rang a midwife, who said wait a bit longer at home when I described what I was feeling. Contractions began soon after this, starting off every 10 minutes or so, then going down to 5 minutes by 12.30, which is when we decided to go back to the hospital.

My hospital had two labour wards: one low-tech, with birthing pools, for low-risk births; the other one high-tech for women having epidurals and caesarians etc. I was quite fit during pregnancy and had wanted an active birth – upright, squatting and labouring in water. However, the contractions had become so intense by the time we got to the low-tech unit that all I wanted to do was lie on my side on the bed.

Around 3pm we were told that because there was a midwife shortage that day, everyone on our ward would have to transfer to the high-tech ward downstairs. I wasn't too upset at having to transfer, but I knew I couldn't stand, let alone walk down the stairs. I remember being taken in the lift with others from the ward, with me the only one in a wheelchair.

Once we were on the medical ward I immediately started on gas and air. Fred was patting my forehead with a damp cloth – he was also having to use it for himself, rather overwhelmed by the occasion. Holding my hand, he encouraged me to focus on breathing, but it was difficult. We were both watching the monitor readings and I realised that the monitor did not seem to reflect what I was feeling. I could see the numbers going up to 50, 60, then down again, but to me the contractions seemed to be more constant than coming and going in peaks and troughs. I was supposed to stop using the gas and air in between contractions, but I couldn't work out where the difference was, apart from what the monitor was saying. I finished a whole canister of gas and air, and had to have a second.

During this time, my midwife and a student had been popping in and out. I had never met them before, but the midwife was very experienced and reassuring and although I was in great pain I felt completely safe throughout. My waters broke while she was checking how dilated I was – there was a sudden deluge onto the bed, wetting my socks.

A while later, I felt that I just couldn't bear the constant pain any longer and said to Fred that I wanted an epidural. He went to find the midwife, who immediately examined me but said it was too late for an epidural, that I was about 8cm dilated. I was not too upset, in fact quite relieved, when she said this. I had known in advance that an epidural might change the course of labour and had hoped that I wouldn't need one, so it was probably a good thing that the decision was taken out of my hands. Also, I knew it wouldn't be long now.

Then all of a sudden I needed to push. Barely able to speak, I sort of gasped "Fred, I need to push now". His reply was "hang on, I'll get the midwife". It took perhaps just a couple of minutes while he found the midwife and she checked me, but they were unbearable minutes, trying to hold back on the urge to push, and I was utterly relieved when she said it was ok for me to go ahead. Then I really pushed – it was painful, but so good to be doing something active. The pain was no longer something happening to me; I was now in control. I reached down to feel the head and was amazed at the feel of it – this is my child, I thought, and all I have to do is push it out of my body. The last two pushes were with every ounce of strength left in my body, and suddenly the baby slid out.

My memory is a blur at this point, until the moment the baby was in my arms wrapped in a blanket. I saw the head and hair first, which were all greasy, wet and bloody; then I smelt the baby, immediately struck by the idea that it was a really familiar smell (like me?); I saw her hands; then finally her face. Fred told me that we had a little girl."

Baby Maya was born after an eight-hour labour.

NICKY'S STORY
Elective caesarian

"During pregnancy I enquired about having an elective caesarian. The reason for this is because when I was a medical student I had attended some births and seen the agony of difficult labours. I didn't want to risk a long, drawn-out labour and to start off motherhood feeling too burnt out to enjoy the baby. My husband is a doctor, and knew some of the obstetricians at the NHS hospital I was booked into, including one of the country's top surgeons who does both private and NHS work. He is well-known in the medical profession for his skill with caesarians – other doctors like to watch him cutting through the layers with precision, and the recovery time for women he's operated on is relatively quick. He offered to do the operation if I wanted it, at 38 weeks.

I am aware of the implications – healthwise and political – of elective caesarians, and I was still not totally decided in the last trimester whether I wanted to try out labour or not. However, when late tests revealed that the baby wasn't growing too well and might have to be induced early anyway, my mind was made up to have the elective caesarian. A few days before the date of the operation I had a show as well, so my baby was clearly ready to be born.

I did get nervous as I was being prepared for the operation and started to tremble uncontrollably. I was given a spinal block and they hooked the sheet up. I felt tugging, but no pain. My husband, being a medical man, couldn't resist looking at the other side of the curtain, and telling me what was going on. The minutes just after the birth itself are a bit confused in my memory. I didn't particularly want to hold my new baby, and was happier to watch her in my husband's arms. Then I did want to hold her and didn't let go for hours – I was like a tigress in my rush of protectiveness over her.

I suffered no pain at all from birth, either during the operation or afterwards. Unlike many women I know who had to have caesarians after being in labour, I was up and walking around within a day, owing to the skill of the surgeon. Breastfeeding was the only thing that turned out to be painful. But I believe strongly in the health benefits of breastfeeding and consider any nipple pain to be worth putting up with, whereas the pain of labour would not have been worthwhile at all."

Baby Poppy was born in 15 minutes. See also pp133 and 204.

MELISSA'S STORY
Water birth

"Having learnt a lot about active birth, I was keen to go through labour with as little intervention as possible. I considered a home birth, but didn't have the confidence to do this with a first labour, so booked into the local hospital, which had a birthing pool.

I was working on my MA dissertation right up until the day before I was due. Richard and I celebrated this with wine, reasoning that it wouldn't hurt the baby at this stage. He went to bed a bit drunk, whereas I started to feel crampy at 1.30am and thought that the wine may have kick-started labour. I decided not to wake up Richard and ran a bath with lavender oil. I wallowed in this through the night, as the cramps slowly got worse. Eventually, at about 6am, I thought I had better wake Richard, who was a bit groggy.

My antenatal teacher had suggested waiting until I felt the need to shout before going into hospital – I started feeling this by around 9.30am. We took a TENS machine and birthing ball in with us in case the birthing pool was not available, but luckily the pool was free. My intention was to labour in the water, but I didn't know whether I wanted to actually deliver in water. I had seen a TV programme showing a water birth, which was quite reassuring – the babies didn't need to breathe immediately and are ok for five minutes underwater. The midwife on duty said she knew how to deliver babies in water.

An examination showed me to be 3cm dilated, and the midwife estimated that I would be in labour for another ten hours. I was violently sick. The contractions had changed pace by now and quite soon I started needing gas and air. Other than that, the pain was about bearable, probably because I was in water – I could stretch out and arch my back, weightless. I didn't invite Richard into the water, though – he was snack monitor, feeding me five crunchy bars and 3 or 4 litres of water during the labour. I would stand up in the pool occasionally between contractions while the two midwives assigned would listen to the baby's heartbeat.

I went through a canister of gas and air and became agitated when no-one could find the porter who had the keys to the cupboard holding the spare canisters. But another examination showed I was in transition and nearly ready to push. It had taken just three hours instead of ten to be fully dilated. The two midwives who had been with me constantly until now were nearing the end of their shift but decided to stay. The two new midwives joined us, then a third who wanted to see a water birth – by now I felt that I couldn't leave the water. The second stage took ages, nearly two hours, but was not too awful. The baby's head came out and was underwater for couple of minutes, then with the next contraction came the shoulders, then the body sort of swam out, and the midwife brought the baby to the surface. We had a girl, and I felt euphoric."

Baby April was born about five hours after proper contractions began.

Charlotte's Story
Two weeks overdue and hoping for a natural birth

"My contractions started at 6am, so fortunately I'd had a good night's sleep. This was to stand me in good stead; I got 10 minutes' sleep in the next 48 hours, and for obvious reasons would not sleep properly for another five months! The old wives' (or modern wives') tale of "curry and sex" seemed to work for a baby who was two weeks late…

The Hours of Labour

The contractions became closer over the next 12 hours, and we went to the hospital around 6pm, when they were about five minutes apart. They were pretty strong by this time and would stop me in my tracks. Once at the hospital, three hours or so passed with little change. I asked for a bath to be run (the only birthing pool was already in use). In between contractions I still felt normal, though rather like a spare part – I was waiting for this big moment, yet I felt fine and as if all the attention on me was somehow misplaced. While the bath was running I took a homeopathic remedy – *caullophyllum* – designed to speed up contractions. This was a bad move: the moment I took this pill, the contractions accelerated to an unbearable level. I never did get into that bath: the gaps between the contractions were too brief even to get out of my pyjama top.

The intensity continued, and I soon knew that I needed an epidural. This took a long time to administer, because I was unable to lie still. Once in, the relief was immediate. For the next four hours the contractions felt minuscule, though I could see on the monitor when I was having them. But the labour made no progress. As the drug started to wear off, I asked for it to be topped up: I was very scared of returning to the same state as before I had entered second stage. Heeding the midwife's instructions to push as every contraction came on, I pushed and pushed and pushed, but with the numbing epidural could feel nothing: I would fill my lungs with air and squeeze down, but couldn't feel where my efforts were aimed.

I carried on like this for an hour-and-a-half, which was exhausting. I'd been on the go now for nearly 24 hours. A senior midwife was called in to discuss breaking my waters: they were still intact, and from my NCT class I had learned that it was perfectly feasible to give birth this way, and that I should resist pressure to have them broken artificially. Obedient to the NCT, I resisted, much to the irritation of the midwives, who clearly thought I was being silly and had learned some claptrap from this middle-class right-on class. I bargained to be given another half hour of pushing. No progress, so they broke my waters. Still no progress after another hour, so a delegation of consultants and whatevers came in, huffing and puffing about ventouse. The baby was showing no signs of distress, so I was anxious still to try to deliver her on my own, but I'd been in second stage for so long that the staff were getting twitchy. I was wheeled off, fighting back tears of exhaustion, disappointment and panic, to theatre, where ventouse was tried unsuccessfully. Amid the glare of lights, with my legs in stirrups and my morale in tatters, my beautiful baby daughter was finally born at 10.40am, by forceps."

Baby Beatrice was born after a 28-hour labour. Charlotte's descriptions of labour pain and her feelings afterwards are on pp27, 35, 56 and 72.

A Closer Look at Labour Pain

Descriptions of labour are usually presented either purely in clinical terms or tending towards the metaphorical. We hear of the various stages of labour. We perhaps form the impression of a battle between the bodies of mother and child, or we subscribe to the active birth metaphor of ocean waves. This section looks at the pain of labour from various angles.

THE STAGES OF LABOUR
Effacement – the cervix pulls flat, and you may have a show (discharge of the mucus plug in cervix). The process can take many days, perhaps unnoticed.

First stage – once your cervix is about 3cm dilated, with contractions coming at least once every five minutes, labour is said to be established. The cervix dilates to a diameter of about 10cm. It could take anything from half an hour to several days. An average seems to be about 12 hours for a first labour.

Second stage – the baby comes through the birth canal. May be five minutes or a couple of hours.

Third stage – the placenta is delivered.

A Universal Experience?

In some cultures, women appear to have quite a strong empathy with each other in the experience of childbirth – pain is openly acknowledged; midwifery skills are held in high regard; newly delivered mothers are cosseted by other women for a month perhaps. But empathy seems to be relatively muted in our own culture. On the whole, labour is a surprisingly taboo subject beyond an acknowledgement of "it will be painful". Medical teachings about labour tend simply to describe the clinical stages (see left panel) and the forms of pain relief that are available (see p56), which are not very enlightening about the actual experience of labour. Then from active birth enthusiasts we glean the idea that with a positive attitude to pain and the opportunity to move about as we want during labour, we will have a more fulfilling birth experience than if we passively allow medical interventions or request artificial relief from pain.

There's perhaps nothing wrong with any such contrasting views *per se*, but unfortunately we now appear to feel more competitiveness than empathy with each other. As with many things relating to motherhood, we tend to compare ourselves with other women, or what we think applies to other women. There is a concept about "pain thresholds". Here are two examples:

"I do sometimes feel a bit of a show-off about my labour: first baby, only seven hours, and just gas and air! In a way I feel proud of my body and a bit of an earth mother. The hospital staff all commented that I had a very high pain threshold, but I don't think this is the case, we all experience pain differently. Other people did seem to have a tougher time than me" (Julia).

"My pain threshold turned out to be lower than I thought and lower than other women's – perhaps because the pain was in the back" (Emma).

Because of the mix of taboo, clinical terminology and spurious comparison, new mothers often feel isolated in their experience of childbirth, despite the fact that they have undergone the same process as countless other women. But that is not to say that we all experience the same thing. Most of the rest of this section focuses on the vast differences in women's experiences of labour pain, which shows why the concept of pain thresholds – and therefore any competitive feelings about succeeding or failing to give birth with minimal relief – is completely ridiculous.

Anatomy of a Contraction

The uterus is an organ of thick muscle with an elongated opening at the cervix. Apparently, it contracts a lot throughout our lives to help blood flow. Usually we can't feel these flexings, but they become more forceful towards the end of pregnancy, as "Braxton Hicks" contractions. In the final days of pregnancy (or under the influence of synthetic hormones for induction), the cervix starts to pull back and flatten out under the force of these contractions. As it starts to dilate, the spasms may become more obvious, and medical people might refer to them as "tightenings" or "twinges". The sensation at this stage varies from period-like cramps to a band of pain lasting for many seconds. Once the cervix has dilated to 3cm, labour is said to be established. The contractions often become heavier, of longer duration, and usually closer together, every few minutes. In full flow, a uterine contraction might begin, imperceptibly for the first 20 seconds or so, continue to build over another half minute, peak, then slowly relax over another half minute. The sensation is mainly focused around the cervix rather than across the whole uterus.

The editor asked some women to describe contractions. For Charlotte they were a combination of pain and an overwhelming feeling of pressure. Caroline said it was a force gathered in a deep part of her body where she had barely had any sensation before, and it literally took her breath away. Anja compared the feeling to someone tormenting her with a huge Chinese burn every time she moved, not something her own body was doing. She forgot that there was a baby in there.

Unquantifiable Pain

Obstetric monitors can measure the strength and length of contractions – if you are hooked up to one at some stage, you might be surprised to find it registering contractions that you cannot feel. The monitors prove that contractions vary in intensity and duration in different labours, and that the level at which they become apparent varies. What opens the cervix with relatively little force in one woman will be the lower end of the scale for another.

DEALING WITH A CHANGE IN GEAR
Many women find they can cope for many hours with a certain level of contractions, but feel alarmed and disorientated when they intensify.

With reassurance and support (especially from a skilled midwife), it is often possible to get a "second wind". On the other hand, a change in gear might herald a decision to start using pain relief, especially if many more hours of labour are anticipated. Just see how it goes on the day!

A Closer Look at Labour Pain

But being able to quantify the intensity of contractions on a monitor is only a small part of the story. What such monitors cannot measure is the debilitating effect of labour as time passes. There is no way of monitoring how much adrenaline and pain-relieving endorphins your brain is triggering. Nor can any other labour-related pains be measured on a monitor, such as the constant lower backache of a "back labour" (when the baby's position is awkward, pressing against your lower back). Claudia, Rosalyn and Caroline all noticed that the monitor did not correspond to their experience – the pain started to become more constant than the peaks and troughs shown on screen. After enduring constant pain for a time, with little or no respite in between contractions, each begged for an epidural. Claudia was 8cm dilated at this stage, six hours from the onset of labour, and advised not to have one; Rosalyn and Caroline were just 3–4cm at this stage, 12 hours and four hours into labour respectively, and grateful for an epidural to be administered.

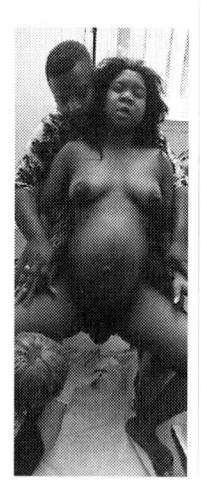

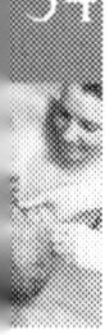

Here are two contrasting anecdotes about labour pain, which show how widely variable the experience can be.

"I think I must be a bit odd, but I didn't find labour that painful. All through my pregnancy I kept reading and hearing descriptions of the pain of labour, but when it came about it was not too bad. One thing that helped was knowing that each contraction was going to end, and that I could have a break. I had bad pain associated with a kidney disorder in the past, which was far worse than labour. I think an understanding of the process of labour and what is happening to your body is an important part of being able to relax into and so overcome pain. I knew why I was hurting and that it wouldn't last for ever" (Julia).

"I got a good breathing rhythm going for a long time, a few hours. But then I got really tired. The contractions intensified, and I was examined and shown to be just 3cm. It was revolting after that, like being tortured. The contractions started coming really close together, and I could barely breathe. I remember groaning and grimacing while kneeling on the bed clinging onto the frame. It was by far the worst experience of my life" (Anja).

Transition and the Pushing Stage

As you near full dilation, and your baby begins to descend, your body might start to tremble and go through great swings in temperature. Vomiting and losing any sense of rhythm with contractions are described by some women. Fortunately, the second stage is usually a matter of minutes when compared with the many hours of contractions that can lead up to full dilation. As the baby's head descends from the uterus, the first part of the mother's body to feel the pressure is

GLORIOUS PAIN?
One way of viewing labour is as a rite of passage. With this view, then you might consider that Nature has given the pain a purpose – humbling you as a woman while at the same time making you mentally stronger for the experience. On the other hand, labour might highlight the savagery of the natural world and leave you craving the world of technology and obstetric assurance. It's not impossible to subscribe to both views at once.

the anus. As the baby's head "crowns", there is likely to be a sensation of being stretched. Most women seem to find that this is unpleasant, but their urge to push overwhelms any other consideration at the time.

Jane S. did not feel the need to use any artificial form of pain relief during the 12 or so hours of her first stage, but described the second stage as "a really horrible physical urge that took over everything else." Hilary had a more graphic description: "I'm sorry to be blunt, but pushing a baby out is like trying to shit a melon. I've had four children and I've found I can cope ok with the contractions, but I've hated the pushing stage each time. It always seems to take ages, probably because my muscles are weak." However, Diana had a very different perspective, having delivered a 10lb baby without needing an episiotomy. "I knew I was carrying a large baby in advance and was worried about how she was going to come out. But my midwife said that I wouldn't necessarily tear, and that I could try massaging my perineum with oil for a couple of weeks. I did this and loads of pelvic floor exercises and, on the day, got her out with five big pushes and no tearing at all. It wasn't nice, but a doddle compared to the first stage."

Fear and External Factors

The link between pain and fear is well known. Learning about the process of labour helps to dispel fear, and if you can see an end in sight you might be able to cope better. But many factors can heighten fear during labour: if, for instance, the pain is much worse than expected, or if monitors show signs of a potential problem. Rosalyn became fearful during labour (see p45), even though she had read up on the process: "I was so miserable after the contractions intensified and a backache developed. Gas and air made no difference whatsoever. The pain was shocking, much more than I'd anticipated (and I had thought it might be pretty bad). In my paranoia, I started putting myself in the shoes of my father's mother, who had died giving birth to him in the 1930s, and I felt an affinity with every woman who had died in childbirth in the history of our species. I was surrounded by hospital technology but in the midst of a personal ordeal of pain and fear."

In stark contrast to Rosalyn's paranoia, Annette (see p39) had little fear of the outcome: "I had never experienced pain of such intensity before this, but I felt very calm during the whole experience and trusted the team around me to do whatever was necessary. I felt I coped with the pain, partly by thinking it cannot last for too long – it has to end. I was being induced, and once contractions started I knew it would not be a really lengthy labour. I also thought about my own mother when she was dying of cancer and took strength from remembering her courage in the face of pain. She wasn't able to fight death, but I knew that I would be all right at the end of labour and have a beautiful baby."

MINIMISING DISCOMFORTS DURING LABOUR

• Unless there are complications, spend the early part of labour in the comfort of your own home rather than in hospital.

• Concentrate on breathing – this can help at any stage.

• Change position every now and then, whether from standing to squatting, sitting or lying down. For example, if you are experiencing back pain, try leaning forwards so the weight of the baby shifts.

• Wallowing in a bath or birthing pool can alleviate some of the weight and pressure in your uterus.

A Closer Look at Labour Pain

Pain is not just about what is happening inside your abdomen. The things going on around you can affect your perception. For example, putting active birth principles into practice is not always possible when you are in a stressful situation. The use of continuous monitoring, which inhibits movement, is a contentious issue because of this. Furthermore, the reaction and support from people around you can affect your state of mind. Unfortunately, in these days of midwife shortages, you may spend many hours labouring in isolation of one-to-one professional support, which is why you must have a labour companion.

Pain Relief

Pain of any sort can take the breath away. When we are scared, the instinct might be to scream and take short little breaths at the top of the lungs. But the body actually needs more oxygenation, not less, when the large muscle that is your uterus starts contracting. Getting a good breathing rhythm going, involving deliberately deep in-breaths and extra long out-breaths will keep your body oxygenated and also give you something on which to focus. Some people chant or hum. Moving around and trying out different ways of sitting and leaning against objects and shifting your weight as the hours of labour go by can also be a good way of "riding the contractions". This sort of thing is the essence of active birth principles. For some women, focusing on breathing is all they need to deal with pain; for others it makes no more than a marginal difference.

Duration of labour is perhaps the most obvious factor in the need for relief. Most of us are able to withstand pain for a while in the same way as we are all able to run for a while. But some of us would be shattered after a few miles of jogging and even the very fittest of us cannot run marathon after marathon. A woman experiencing powerful contractions is obviously going to crave relief as her body tires, whether that is in two hours or 20 from the onset of labour. The body will tire even if contractions are mild but taking place over more than the course of a day, as it would if you were walking in all that time without rest.

All forms of artificial pain relief have their pros and cons, so it's best to learn about them in advance. But don't fall into the trap of deciding in advance how you want to "manage" labour (see pp34 and 71). As this section shows, the duration of labour and intensity of contractions are not absolutes or reliable indications of difficulty. Keep your options open throughout.

Nine in ten women try some form of artificial pain relief. Julia had a straightforward labour (see pp38–39) and says "I found that using gas and air combined with breathing techniques learnt in yoga, I was able to set up a rhythm to ride each contraction." Ruth tried several forms: "I'd done the breathing

ARTIFICIAL RELIEF
• *A portable TENS machine. This sends electrical pulses through pads to block some of the pain in early labour. But it can be expensive and possibly of little use once labour is established.*

• *Gas and air canisters are available in maternity units and can be brought to your home. It leaves only a short-term residue in you and your baby. But it is only partial relief.*

• *Pethidine and other opiates can be given by a midwife. As with gas and air, they provide partial relief, but can cause nausea. They leave a longer residue in you and your baby.*

• *Epidural – see p21.*

The Hours of Labour

exercises, I'd even gone to yoga, but the pain was far worse than any breathing or change of position could deal with. The contractions were bearable for about three or four hours, then after that the pain took my breath away and reduced me to tears. I was very relieved to be given pethidine, which was lovely and dreamy for a while. But then the pain started to get even worse and they needed to induce me to speed up labour, so an epidural was given. That was better than the pethidine – total pain relief, yet I could still walk and move around."

Charlotte tried various methods, too: "I coped with mild contractions for many hours, with deep breathing and a TENS machine. Then they accelerated to an unbearable level. Gas and air provided little relief. Likewise the TENS machine by this stage, whose wires ended up driving me mad, and which I tore off mid-contraction. The gap between the contractions was so short that I couldn't stay still long enough for the anaesthetist to administer the epidural. I was desperate for this magical drug, and in the end my husband lay on top of me to keep me still enough for the anaesthetist to do his job. The relief was immediate."

Feelings After the Event

When they come to reflect on the great event afterwards, some women find that the memory of the pain and how they reacted to it arouses feelings of either pride or failure. Both Ruth and Rosalyn were grateful for medical intervention but also disappointed with their own bodies. Rosalyn often thinks about what labour must have been like for women in the days before epidurals and life-saving equipment. Ruth says, "I can't begin to imagine what the pain would have been like without the drugs. I had an obstructed labour and would have died in other circumstances – i.e. not a "natural" mother. I've no doubt that it is different for different women. No-one should feel bad about taking drugs. You have no idea before you start whether you will be delivering in three hours or 36."

But another factor that might play on the mind after birth is that labour might have taken a different course if no pain relief were used. Epidurals can slow down contractions, and the loss of sensation at the pushing stage can lead to the need for ventouse or forceps, or even a caesarian. Thus, feelings of relief about the benefits of an epidural might be offset by regret.

The most positive thing about birth is, of course, the baby itself. The majority of us start to forget about the ordeal within a matter of weeks (see also pp71–73). We all deserve praise for getting through birth, no matter what the details, and the greatest reassurance and regard should go to those who experience long, difficult labours. Now all we have to do is recover and look after the child… the rest of this book is devoted to how we do that…

SO WHY DON'T WE ALL HAVE ELECTIVE CAESARIANS? Unless there is a complication with labour and vaginal delivery, caesarian carries a slightly higher risk to maternal health and often takes longer to recover from than a straight-forward vaginal birth.

The baby has to come out one way or the other – for the majority of women the ideal way is vaginally, for some it is abdominally. If you are like the editor, you fear both ways, but are willing to go through the ordeal – whatever it involves – in order to have the child you long for.

THE FIRST DAYS TOGETHER

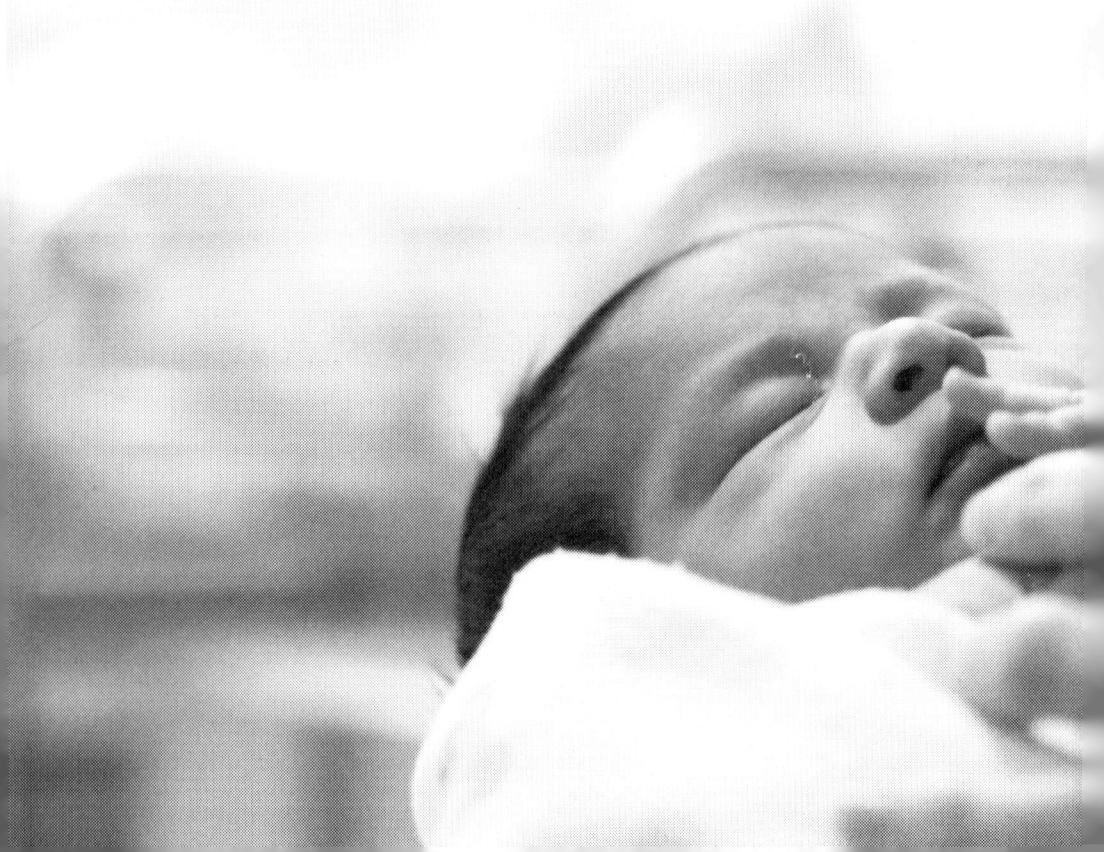

59

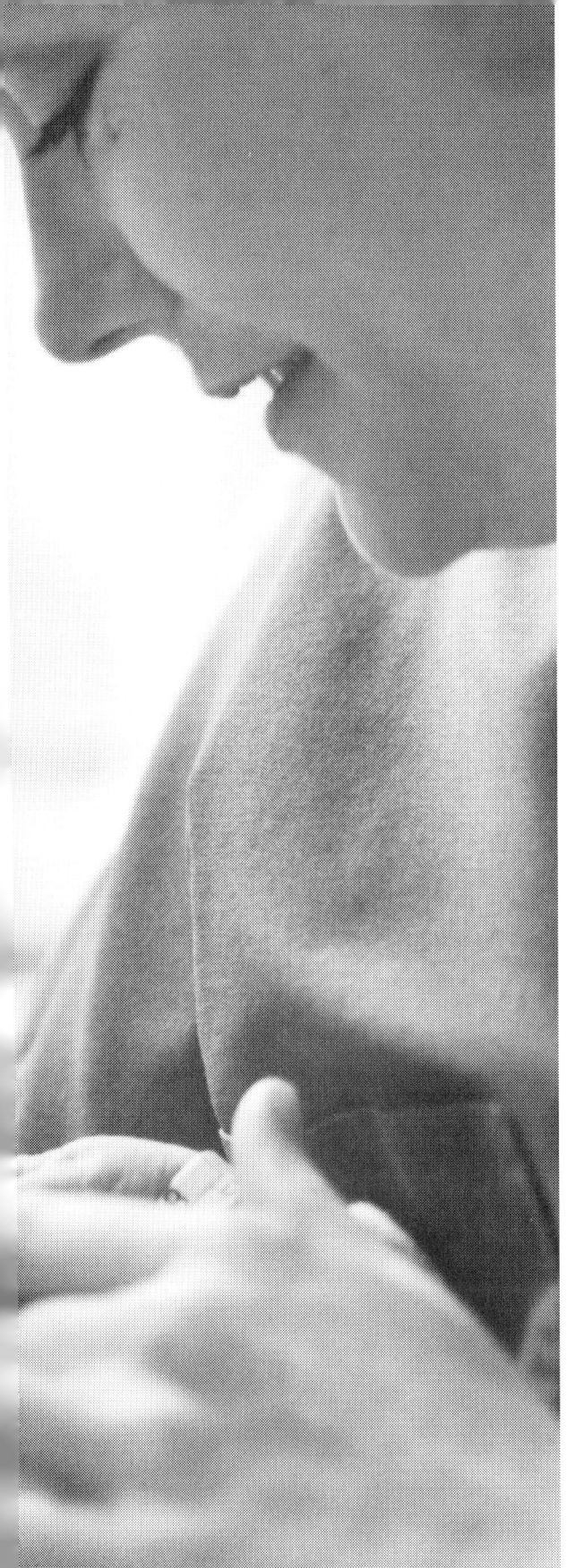

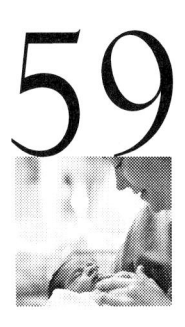

Contents

60 Stories of the First Hours

62 Life on the Postnatal Ward

66 Physical Discomforts

68 Going Home and Support at Home

71 When You Have to Find a Way Through Trauma

Stories of the First Hours

With the heavings of birth over and done with, and your baby taking lungfuls of air and a look at the world outside your body, your first hours of motherhood might be a mixture of relief, amazement, wonder, weariness and trepidation.

First Interactions

Many parents describe a sense of surprise, shock and wonder when they first meet their child. For some, it is a positive feeling; for others, it is one of ambivalence. Following a long, hard labour, the natural response might be just to want to "shut down" and put off dealing with "the creature" until you've had some sleep. Some people describe a love at first sight – this is looked at on p203. Perhaps most of us do not fall in love immediately. By contrast, the first feeds and dressing your new baby are among the practical ways in which you start to build your intense, personal relationship together.

Amy gave birth at home and felt utterly overwhelmed in the first minutes after birth. "I was kneeling, and after endless pushing, the baby whooshed out, a dark, bloody mess onto the floor. I was trembling and didn't want to look closely at what had come out for a while. Everyone else seemed so excited. The baby just lay on the floor screeching. I think the others were waiting for me to react – to pick up and cuddle and say something significant, I suppose. I was so relieved when the midwife took the initiative to cut the cord, clean up and wrap the baby in a blanket and pass to me to hold whilst she dealt with the placenta. I think I said "oh my god" and "look at you" a few times. It was ages, maybe half an hour, before I even thought to look at whether I had a boy or a girl."

Justine had been in labour for three days (see p41). "My first thought when she popped out between my thighs – how could something so big come out of me?! I expected her to be wrinkly and mis-shapen, but she was plump and rosy cheeked, with blonde curls, big blue eyes, long eyelashes, perfect oval nails... I couldn't believe how beautiful she was. When she fed was the first time she felt real." Caroline was also surprised at the size of her baby and "amazed by the life force in one so young." Emma thought that her new son had a "very true stare and looked far wiser than a newborn." Teresa hardly dared to look into the face of the child she had been carrying for nine months.

The First Days Together

Some women recall certain moments or feelings, but don't remember the exact order. After a forceps delivery (see p45), Rosalyn recalls a baby with an ethereally beautiful face and the sound of lustful crying. "Someone said it was a girl and I announced the name we wanted, Minna Rose. I asked my boyfriend to hold her while I threw up. Somehow the placenta was removed without me seeing it at all, to my regret. I may even have fainted or swooned for a bit. I was happier to watch my boyfriend holding the baby rather than hold her myself, but I also remember feeding her for the first time while we were still in the labour room, and being amazed that she automatically knew what to do. The three of us were left alone to doze for a few hours. Then I was taken in a wheelchair to a postnatal room, with various tubes still attached."

First Time Alone

At some stage on the first day you will probably be left alone with your baby to rest together. Far from getting rest, though, this might be a time of awe and perhaps trepidation at the immense responsibilities you have for this new life. Annette had this feeling after her fast induction (see p39). "Once I was taken up to the ward and settled into my room, and Tony finally went home, Annie and I were left together and suddenly there was nobody else except her and me. I held her and just could not believe that she was finally here, and that Tony and I had made this beautiful little girl together."

It was the middle of the night when Julia (see p38) arrived on the postnatal ward. "We were told that David would have to leave once we were settled. The midwife left and drew the curtains around us. We were alone at last; it seemed very calm and peaceful. Caitlin fed a bit and dozed in my arms. She was so perfect. Three hours later an exhausted David decided to go home and get some sleep. The hospital staff had not chucked him out as they had said they would. All night I gazed at my daughter – I couldn't sleep. In the morning I fed her and thought I'd better change her nappy, but I wasn't sure how. Anyway, I managed, and was really pleased with myself."

Ruth had a very hard labour (see p40). "I was so tired and weak, I couldn't hold Rosa, but just gazed at her in her cot. I do remember feeling relieved initially, and then for a period of a few hours, feeling panic strike, that I'd made a terrible mistake and couldn't take care of this baby."

For Tina, the first few hours were nightmarish. "Olivia had a low Apgar score and had to go to the neonatal unit. I was transferred to the postnatal ward, and crashed out on the bed, crying. No-one came to see me for two hours – Tim had gone back home by then. It was terrible hearing other mothers and babies behind curtains, and not having my own." (See Tina's story on p73.)

Life on the Postnatal Ward

For the vast majority of women in Britain, the first days with their new baby are spent on the postnatal ward of an NHS hospital. The average length of stay varies around the country, from less than 24 hours in London to three or four days in Scotland, or perhaps a week in the aftermath of a caesarian or complications.

BENEFITS OF BEING ON A POSTNATAL WARD
• Immediate medical attention in the event of complications.
• Health advice and general support in the early days of motherhood.

DISADVANTAGES
• You are in an institutional public setting.
• Your partner cannot share all the experiences or take much responsibility in the early days.

A Typical NHS Postnatal Ward

For the majority of mothers, birth and the days that follow are the first time they have ever spent as a hospital in-patient, which can be an experience in itself.

NHS hospitals vary in how their postnatal wards are set up. Some have a series of rooms with a few beds in each. Others have just one large room with, say, 20 beds, separated with the standard hospital curtains. A few have some single rooms in addition to the main ward, which might be semi-private – a fee will be charged if you want to use one, subject to availability on the day (you probably cannot book such a room in advance). There will be washroom facilities, showers and toilets on the ward. Some of the single rooms might have their own shower and toilet, or shared with just a few others. Breakfast, lunch and dinner will be served free – there will probably be a choice of dishes, including a vegetarian option. You are allowed to bring in your own food, or for visitors to bring you some. For more on Maternity Facilities see pp12–15.

Unless there are complications, the baby will be given a small cot next to your bed. It may come as a surprise, but you will be expected to care for the baby yourself unless you are very weak after the birth, in which case the midwives can help change, wash and comfort your baby while you rest. You will probably be offered advice on breastfeeding and bathing your baby, and how to care for the umbilical stump, which will have a clamp attached for a few days (usually this just means ignoring it).

The ward sisters and midwives will have a station on or near the ward. Next to your bed will be a button that you can press to call for assistance if you are unable to get out of bed. There should always be at least one midwife on the ward 24 hours a day. The obstetricians (specialist doctors for mothers) and paediatricians (specialist doctors for children) might make their ward rounds once a day, in the morning. These doctors will assess whether you and the baby are healthy enough to be discharged from hospital care. If your baby gets the all-clear from the paediatrician but the obstetrician says that your health is still low, then you will both stay on the ward. However, if you are fine but your baby is ill, then there may be several options, according to hospital policy: you might both remain on the ward; the baby might go to a neonatal unit while you remain on the ward; or the baby might go to a neonatal unit while you go home.

Visiting Hours

Ever since a couple of heavily publicised cases of baby-snatching from hospitals a few years ago, most postnatal wards now have some kind of a security system at the main door, making it more difficult for the general public to enter the ward. CCTV might be installed, too. Visiting hours vary amongst hospitals – from midday to 8pm is fairly typical. Visitors might be limited to two at a time, other children might be banned, or only close relatives might be allowed, so do check hospital policy before inviting people to visit.

Restricted visiting has its pros and cons. The main drawback is that your husband or boyfriend, or other close people cannot be by your side constantly to share the experiences of these early days with your baby, nor to help with the practicalities. If you deliver in the night then your birthing partner will probably have to leave as soon as you transfer to the postnatal ward. On the positive side, the restrictions mean that the postnatal ward is less chaotic outside of visiting hours. One of the main reasons why visiting hours are enforced is not so much from a worry about germs but to ease overcrowding and so make life a bit easier for newly delivered mothers. In exceptional circumstances, such as if there is a sudden health problem in you or your baby, then your visitor might be allowed to stay outside of visiting hours. But try not to be too upset if the rules have to be rigidly enforced.

WHAT TO PACK IN YOUR HOSPITAL BAG
• Old, loose-fitting clothes, breastfeeding bras and breast pads.
• High-absorbency sanitary towels with wings, and cotton knickers (see p66).
• Eye shades, ear plugs, mufflers.
• Wash kit, flannels and bath towels.
• Snack bars and fruit.
• Phonecard for hospital phone system (mobiles interfere with high-tech hospital equipment).

FOR YOUR BABY
• Clothes – all-in-ones are good at this stage.
• "Posset cloths" for mopping up regurgitated milk.
• Nappies and wipes.

Noise

In bygone times, babies were whisked away to a line of cots in a nearby nursery, for the sake of hygiene and peace for the exhausted mothers, but, as widely acknowledged, to the detriment of bonding. Nowadays, hygiene is not considered to be so crucial, whereas bonding, quite rightly, is. So babies now usually stay with their mothers on the postnatal ward. You can cuddle, feed and admire your new baby as much as you want, but, of course, you will be disturbed by your baby crying, along with everyone else's. There is also all the other inevitable hospital noise of people and clatter. Ruth was one of many women to find the noise on the postnatal ward stressful in itself. "It really was very hard to sleep. I had two hours on the first night because they took the baby

Life on the Postnatal Ward

away for observation, but after that I only got an hour here and there until I got home." Jo was in a room with just three other beds, but as soon as one baby woke up crying, hers did too, so she didn't sleep very well. And there was no question of sleeping beyond 7am, because that was when they started to lay out breakfast. "But I doubt if I would have slept much even if I were at home, because he was feeding every two hours to begin with."

Rosalyn had to stay in hospital for ten days, because her blood pressure was still high following delivery, and she needed a blood transfusion. "I didn't sleep at all in that time because of the noise, chaos and stress of the situation. Thank god I was in a separate room for the first five days, although I could still hear nearby women in labour crying and groaning, and the noise of baby heartbeat monitors echoed around the whole time – I still have nightmares about those sounds. On the seventh day I was transferred to the main postnatal ward with 17 other women and babies, and within hours got almost hysterical with all the cacophany and lack of privacy. It was the worst environment I have ever been in, and at the very time when I was craving peace."

Stella's friends had warned her about the noise. "I took wax ear plugs and eyeshades. I could still hear the noise but it was mercifully muffled – to the extent that a midwife had to shake my shoulder because Charlie was crying."

Support on the Ward

In the immediate days following birth, when many things may seem strange and new, and your emotions are perhaps a mix of triumph and terror, midwives on the ward are the people you will naturally turn to for advice and support. At this extraordinary and vulnerable time of our lives, it seems that we often remember our midwives either with great fondness and gratitude, or sadly the opposite, with disappointment and anger. The midwifery profession in the NHS is facing shortages (see p24), and the overworked, underpaid people who choose to be midwives have varying levels of abilities. Some are highly professional and genuinely caring. Others are less so. NHS shortages may also be manifested on postnatal wards in problems of bed availability and facilities. Here are some mothers' anecdotes about the support on the ward.

Ruth was relieved to stay four days on the postnatal ward. "The care was fine, and the midwives were wonderful except that they all have a different technique for breastfeeding, which is not helpful, when you are in pain. I do remember one midwife, on a night shift, who couldn't understand why I was crying so much. I tried to explain (the shock of becoming a mother, trauma of emergency etc), and she looked at me and said "you will never stop crying – I still cry over my son and he's 18!" That played over in my mind for a long time."

DURATION OF STAY
It's worth finding out in advance what the hospital policy is for normal length of stay.

You will probably be advised to stay longer if, for example, you developed pre-eclampsia or some other condition during pregnancy; after a caesarian; there was meconium in the waters or some other infection risk; or you lost a lot of blood during delivery.

Some women who have delivered at home might be asked to go into hospital for a checkup.

The First Days Together

Justine was in a hospital that discharges mothers and babies a few hours after a straightforward birth, but doctors kept them in for 24 hours to check that meconium had not been inhaled by the baby. "I was in a side room, and hardly anyone came to see me, even the food trays bypassed the room. It was so depressing to find that the shower was broken, with just a dribble of tepid water coming out. I was exhausted and didn't know what to do except feed Ella constantly. I eventually rang for a midwife in the early hours as I couldn't understand why Ella was crying so much. The midwife was a bit cross and told me the baby was starving, then left the room. But at least the next day my birth midwives (all three teams!) came in to cuddle my babe and marvel at my quick pushing."

Alice thought that the midwives and nurses did a fantastic job in very difficult circumstances, but says "the doctors were overall less impressive – a couple I encountered were downright offensive in their manner and approach towards me." Liz was positive about the entire support team in her Midlands hospital. "I sent a thankyou card, because they were the most caring and hardworking people I have ever met. My own mother had a worse time in hospital back in the Seventies, but attitudes on the ward have really changed since then." But Nicky felt that attitudes on the ward were still old-fashioned, and that midwives were not supportive enough with breastfeeding.

Rosalyn was in a London hospital with a shortage of staff. "The midwives were the most extraordinary mix of angels and devils. I will always fondly remember the lovely Caribbean midwife called Comfort and the sister who placed my baby at the exact angle for breastfeeding while I lay on my side. Incredible expertise. But there were also a couple of nasty midwives: one of them even pinched my breast – she wanted to see if colostrum was coming out but didn't think to ask my permission or at least give a warning. The level of hygiene was appalling – toilets overflowing with bloody cloths. The impact of the problems in the NHS really hit home."

Georgina was another who found the hospital stay traumatic following her caesarian birth to twins. "It was a constant hubbub of babies crying and midwives shouting. I was so relieved to go home." Elaine discharged herself when she learnt that an amenity room wasn't available. She didn't want to share the precious first days of her new life with 15 other women instead of her husband. She also worried about the baby being abducted – "I'm sure it's an irrational fear, but you fear everything at first". On the other hand, Kirstie was relieved not to be discharged for three days from her Scottish hospital. "I knew nothing about babies, but the midwives showed me how to pick her up, bath her and swaddle, and they didn't make me feel silly for having problems with breastfeeding. I'd have been lost without their support."

Baby Ella has her first bath with a midwife on the postnatal ward. The plastic clip on her umbilical stump will remain for several days.

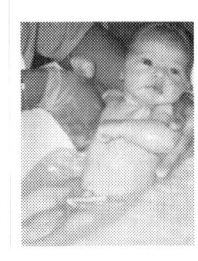

PHYSICAL DISCOMFORTS

There are a number of common physical discomforts in the aftermath of labour. Most ease off within a few days or weeks. Any pain or discomfort that persists beyond the six-week postnatal checkup probably needs specialist treatment – don't suffer in silence.

PERINEAL DISCOMFORT AND LOCHIA

When contemplating an impending birth, most of us worry about how our sensitive perineums are going to fare. Thinking about a 10-cm diameter head squeezing out the vagina or the surgical cut of an episiotomy could make the most courageous of people shiver. It's certainly true that a lot of women experience a degree of soreness in this region in the aftermath of birth. However, the pain might not turn out to be as bad as you feared – out of the women interviewed for this book, only two said they suffered worse discomfort from stitches and tearing than anticipated.

Many women are taken by surprise, however, by weakened bladder and bowel muscles. This is when the pelvic floor exercises taught during antenatal classes come into their own. A few sets of these each day should soon help the three passages – urethra, vagina and anus – back to strength (see panel). But also consult your doctor if you have any incontinence.

Expect the bleeding, called lochia, to continue for several weeks, changing in colour from red to yellowy brown. Don't assume that very heavy bleeding is normal – report it. Having to use towels for weeks on end is a real misery for women who are used to tampons (which are not advisable after birth because of an infection risk). The sanitary towels doled out in hospitals and birth packs tend to be of the old-fashioned mattress variety, sporting descriptions like "maternity strength". In fact, the modern slimline super-strength pads for normal periods are just as absorbent and less uncomfortable. There is also a fashion for buying disposable knickers for the event, which makes sense if your lingerie is all lace and thongs, but standard cotton pants might be more comfortable than voluminous disposables.

Annette had stitches but did not feel a huge amount of discomfort – or at least not as much as she thought there would be. Rosalyn also had stitches and some small broken haemoerrhoids, "but, honestly, they barely hurt at all. Far

---

SELF-HELP FOR THE PELVIC FLOOR
If you feel any weakness in your anus, or you find you are leaking urine or your vagina feels "over-stretched", then you must do loads of pelvic floor exercises. You should have been taught these on antenatal classes, but if not, follow the method below.

Basically, just squeeze your pelvic floor muscles as tight you can and for as long as possible. Imagine you are pulling a tampon up inside you, trying to stop the flow of urine and a bowel movement all at the same time. Hold for as long as you can – which might be anything from two to 20 seconds – then relax. Do a set of, say, ten, every few hours or whenever you remember. You should notice a difference within days.

more upsetting was my anal weakness right after birth. With pelvic floor exercises I got a lot of strength back within a week, although to this day I am a bit weak down there. The bleeding was no worse than a normal period, but dribbled on for weeks – I got sick of the smell of it. Soon after it finished, though, sex was surprisingly good."

To her amazement, Justine had no tearing, but was tender in the region. "I was nervous about doing a poo, and the bleeding was greater than I expected. Yet most surprisingly, I felt quite randy when I saw my partner the day after birth." But any thoughts of physical affection were a long way from Teresa's mind: "The stitches were excruciating for over a week. In fact, I am still annoyed that the hospital stitched me up too tight."

OTHER DISCOMFORTS

Top of the postnatal discomforts table are the debilitating effects of an emergency caesarian. About 20–25% of British mothers will experience the shock to the system of this major abdominal surgery. Discomforts in the caesarian aftermath might include pain around the scar, an inability to move for hours, and a ban on lifting things or driving for some weeks. You will need extra help in hospital and in the early weeks at home (see p155 onwards).

Breastfeeding can be uncomfortable at first (see p114 onwards). Back pain is another common problem. Pregnancy weakens the lower back, birth puts a tremendous strain on it, and poor posture during breastfeeding and while carrying your baby and changing nappies exacerbates any problem. Consult an obstetric physiotherapist (see p15), osteopath or chiropractor if you suffer any back pain after birth – it's more likely to get worse than better if left untreated. An old back injury flared up after Jane's delivery; Rosalyn had compacted vertebrae at the base of her spine after a back labour; and Hilary slipped a disc in heaving herself out of a birthing pool in mid-contraction. Osteopathy helped these three women.

Ruth recalls the miserable aftermath of her caesarian: "I was in abject misery for 24 hours and moderate misery after that for a few weeks. After a caesarian section you are catheterised and on morphine – it's fine until the morphine wears off and the catheter is out. They had warned me that they might have damaged my bladder in the operation by putting a stitch in it by mistake. In fact, they had not, but in any case my bladder and bowel had no real sensation for approximately three weeks. This is normal, apparently, after abdominal surgery. Apart from that, the wound opened up and became infected once I was at home, which was demoralising rather than serious. It took two months to heal. And my nipples felt as though someone had taken a cheese grater to them. But even that got better after two or three weeks."

SOME REMEDIES FOR A SORE PERINEUM

• Taking lots of baths, sitting in a bowl of water to pee, or running a shower over the perineum whilst on the toilet seem to be popular practices.

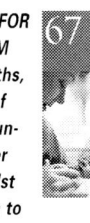

• The Active Birth Centre (p17) sells a herbal sitz bath. It takes ages to prepare, but might help.

• Witch hazel preparations are available from pharmacies.

• Haemoerrhoids (piles) can be alleviated with special creams, available on the postnatal ward or from pharmacies.

Midwives might have other recommendations. Note that surgical stitching has improved since our mothers gave birth. You shouldn't need a special cushion.

Going Home and Support at Home

For the 19 out of 20 British women who give birth in hospital rather than at home, the homecoming is an emotional time. The institutional medical setting is replaced with domestic comforts, but the 24-hour professional help is no longer to hand. Somehow, you will have to muddle through.

Change in Body and Status

The length of time you spend in hospital will depend on how your birth went and where you live in the country. But however long you've been away, and however good, bad or indifferent your experience of hospital was, coming back home with your baby as a separate being rather than as part of your pregnancy heightens the awareness that life has irrevocably changed. Emma said that her house seemed like paradise compared to the cheerless hospital setting, and other mothers have mentioned that their home somehow looked different. For Rosalyn, the grass was literally longer after her 10-day hospital stay.

Alice found that going home was a fantastic but also very strange experience. "I felt like I'd been in hospital for about a month, rather than three nights, and coming out into the sunshine and seeing people out and about doing everyday things made me feel like an alien. That feeling didn't change for several weeks. It is wonderful to introduce your new baby to its home. You do not re-enter your home as the same person you were when you left. When you leave, you are still this "I'm very important because I'm pregnant" person, backed up by a loving partner. When you come back, you're both in a state of shock and totally obsessed with the baby, not yourselves."

Ruth says: "I remember failing to have worked out how to put the car seat in the car in advance. We had to ask someone to help us and were there, outside the hospital, for 20 minutes struggling with seat belts. A passer-by wished us luck with our newborn, and tears came to my eyes. The silence struck us when we got home – no midwives, no medical backup, no camaraderie of a postnatal ward. Just us and this baby. We felt like total amateurs, and that first night she didn't sleep until 4am. I recall feeling euphoric, when, on waking at 7am, I realised that the baby had survived a night in our sole care, and so that was a good start."

SUPPORT FROM OTHER PEOPLE

No new mother should be expected to cope alone with her baby in the early days, especially not if she is recovering from a long labour or a caesarian. Fortunately, many employers are more flexible about paternity leave these days, though it can be used up all too quickly. Close family are the ones who many of us turn to in this time of need. Yet families are sometimes too distant or disparate to be of much practical help, even if good intentions are there. Friends can in turns be a help or hindrance. A typical sound piece of advice is not to have too many visitors, though of course you want to show off the baby.

The standard medical support is that a midwife will visit you at home once a day for the first 10 days after birth. If you are in hospital for a few days then the visits will be proportionately fewer once you get home. After 10 days the care switches to health visitors. An alternative source of professional help is a private maternity nurse, who cares for both mother and child in the early weeks. If you can, arrange help of some sort or another for the early weeks, whether this is from a partner taking extended unpaid paternity leave, family, friends or paid help, even a cleaner to deal with the increased number of chores (more laundry etc).

EUPHORIA AND FEAR *Huge waves of emotion are characteristic of the early post-partum period – these are explored in more detail in Love and Triumph, pp199–213.*

TYPICAL HARDHIPS OF THE EARLY WEEKS

If you are reading this while in the first weeks of parenthood, it might help to know that virtually all new mothers seem to find the early weeks very hard. Don't think of yourself as pathetic or unnatural if the thrill of having a baby is being offset by the down side. (And if you are somehow finding it all very easy, please don't say as such to any other new parent who may be feeling fragile beneath a veneer of bliss.)

Tiredness and weakness are the main hardships, making even the easiest of tasks difficult. Women who had tough, long labours will have a harder time in the early weeks than those whose labours were relatively quick and straightforward. While some mothers are up and about and feeling quite strong within hours of a quick birth, it can literally take up to several months to physically recover from a difficult birth experience.

Hardship comes from being on call 24 hours a day. You wouldn't feel so put out if the newborn baby simply slept and then woke up, happy to wait for a drink of milk, an occasional nappy change and wash, and some cuddles. But babies are far more complex in their needs, and very vocal with them. Their waking lives are a deluge of sensations, instincts and unfathomable emotions, and they wail and shriek at odd hours round the clock. Much of the day and night is spent feeding and comforting a newborn baby. In the early weeks there is so much to do for the baby that there is hardly any window for anything else, so much so that eating supper or taking a bath without disturbance seems like a luxury. It can feel like life has irrevocably slipped beyond control. And parenthood can be a shock, no matter how mentally prepared you try to be before your first birth. There's the dramatic change in status from expectant parent to parent, the sudden weight of responsibility for this helpless human being you created, the bombardment of contradictory advice about good parenting that you have to pick your way through… Perhaps all of us go through emotional turmoil and have unsettling shifts in our sense of self at this time. This is looked at on p232.

Unfortunately, any other major worries you have relating to relationships, finances, career and moving house are even more likely to come to the fore when you have a baby. If you can, though, try to push other such things to one side for now, until you and your baby have both settled into an agreeable rhythm together. For more on this, see the Feeding and Sleeping chapters.

TYPICAL STORIES ABOUT THE EARLY WEEKS

All the women interviewed had found the first month or two either "quite hard" or "very, very hard indeed". Maria said that birth had been easier and less painful than she had been expecting, but dealing with colic left her feeling ragged. Justine found weeks three to six almost unbearable. "Ella had a "growing spurt" and fed nearly continuously from 6am till midnight. When she wasn't eating she was crying. I desperately needed sleep, my back ached from carrying her, my nipples were sore. Everyone said the first six weeks are the hardest and they are." Yet, as Justine pointed out, this period also coincides with a baby's first smiles.

Annette found that her sister and some close friends were extremely supportive when her husband went back to work, but at such a poignant time she missed her own mother, who had died a few years earlier. The midwives who visited were in turns helpful or in a great rush. "Fortunately, I did not find Annie too difficult in the first few weeks, but I did feel quite emotional for no particular reason and I hadn't realised how tiring breastfeeding would be."

Ruth and Rosalyn had to recover from major health problems, but were saved by having boyfriends at home who looked after them for weeks. "He did everything," said Ruth, "breakfast in bed, not to mention lunch, tea and dinner, and he took the baby away and let me sleep for two hours. In fact I remember those early weeks as being in a cocoon. It took about three months before the exhaustion and pain from the birth had subsided." The single mothers interviewed had all sought help from their families at this time, except Mariko, whose family and former friends abroad had ostracised her for having a child outside marriage. "Women like me have to be tougher than soldiers," she said.

FATHERS IN THE EARLY WEEKS
Especially with the modern emphasis on exclusive breastfeeding, fathers can feel alienated in the early weeks. They might be expected to go back to work within days, feeling burdened by responsibility. Childbirth, more than any other aspect of life, divides the sexes and exposes inequalities between men and women, which can be another difficult issue in the early weeks. But many mothers would still cite the father as the main person from whom they want moral support.

When You Have to Find a Way Through Trauma

Bringing a new person into the world has the potential for high drama. To be born and to give birth are among our most dangerous moments in life, and some of us feel a brush with mortality in the process. If events take an unexpected and alarming turn, the emotional after-effects can run deep.

Births That Don't Go "To Plan"

If there's one thing pregnant women should really avoid (above soft cheese and an extra glass of wine), it's building idealised expectations about birth. It's good to look into various options and know in advance the benefits and disadvantages of different methods of pain relief and medical interventions. But to "set your heart", as some of us seem to do, on a birth without medical intervention is losing sight of what can be at stake. The natural birth movement has done a lot of good, but unfortunately has also brought in, for some women, the emotional trauma of "failing" to have a natural birth. The encouragement to make "birth plans" (see p34) can lead to idealisation – if you do write a plan, make sure you don't set it in stone. The fact of the matter is, you cannot predict how long labour is going to last, nor what might crop up along the way, and the odds are actually loaded against a first birth going entirely smoothly. Putting active birth principles into practice is one thing, feeling that you should endure the whole of labour without artificial relief for the sake of doing it naturally is quite another.

Alice had planned a drug-free water birth, but after several days of labour ended up with a caesarian (see her story on p41). These are her reflections on the experience: "Childbirth is definitely traumatic to some degree. Mine was extremely upsetting because it was so different from my expectations. Also, I think it's really important to recognise how traumatic childbirth can be for the father. At least the woman has something to "do", but all the partner can do is watch and try to mentally cope with what he's seeing. My partner went home a few hours afterwards, where the enormity of the whole thing hit him. Meanwhile, I was handed a baby to start looking after, so I didn't really have a chance to think or reflect on the trauma at the time. Later, the two of us were able to deal with the negative feelings by talking honestly about them. Without doing that, I'm not sure how one can otherwise deal with trauma."

Charlotte experienced great pain during a long labour (pp50–51), and her daughter was eventually born with the aid of forceps: "In retrospect I rather regret having made a birth plan. For me, everything ended up going contrary to the plan, so I felt endless disappointment. Also, in my naivety, I had invested the labour and birth with all sorts of positive images, and for me there was nothing positive about it except the very end result: that my baby emerged, unharmed and beautiful. I have a friend whose baby was born two days after mine. Her labour was virtually identical and in some ways more difficult (she was transferred from a cottage hospital to a main one in the middle of labour), yet she wasn't traumatised by the event. I am sure that the fact that she read very little beforehand, made no birth plan, and is a nurse – and hence used to hospital routines – all helped make her experience more positive. Another friend, whose baby was born at home, was in labour for three days, yet didn't find it traumatic. My labour, for whatever reasons, was intensely uncomfortable, and I would be reluctant to go through the same experience again, despite the fact that I adore my baby and am immensely proud of her and of myself."

Labour Dramas

Most women experience pain during labour – and of course any painful situation can leave an emotional residue. On top of that, an emergency or even the merest hint of a problem for your baby or you during the event is likely to be traumatic. The emergency may be resolved quickly at the time, but the way in which you mentally replay the birth afterwards might centre on the most terrifying moment. For instance, if the baby shows signs of distress (often shown by a dramatic change in heart rate), various forms of intervention might be used to hasten birth. The baby might recover quickly, but the fear of the moment and the nature of the intervention might play on your mind for some time. Post-traumatic stress disorder has been diagnosed in some women following a difficult birth.

On the other hand, the mind usually deals with trauma such as this by fading the memory out after it has been replayed a number of times. It seems that most women half forget the exact nature of any labour dramas within a few weeks, and certainly by a few months, especially if they aren't carrying any misplaced sense of guilt or shattered expectations about birth. Ruth's stories about her dramatic birth and its aftermath are on pp40, 61, 63, 67 and 68. She says: "I remember wishing I had the space and time to have a good weep and recover from the emergency operation. But you just don't have time. It's only recently that I've looked back and realised that the whole experience was extremely frightening. When the curtain was pulled away after the caesarian, the two surgeons were covered in blood, like something out of a film. But the memories do fade. If I get pregnant again, then I will probably feel more frightened of the birth, but right now, seven months later, it's not traumatic."

Health Problems Following Birth

Breathing difficulties or infection in the baby, or anaemia from blood loss in the mother are perhaps more common than people realise. Jaundice in the baby is quite common – mentioned by several parents interviewed. Usually jaundice is mild, and perhaps all you have to do is hold the child up to daylight. But some parents have major worries over health in the days following birth.

Tina and Tim's daughter, Olivia, was born with lung problems. Tina describes feelings of horror at seeing her child "stuck with tubes, like a pin cushion". She stayed one night, but being on the ward without her baby was unbearable, so she went home while Olivia stayed. "We were numb," says Tina. "I would express milk with a machine and take it in to be fed through a tube in her nose – no-one imagines a scene like that when they dream about having a baby. But seeing twins in the neonatal unit who were half the size of Olivia, yet doing ok, gave me hope."

Olivia came home after two weeks. Then Tina was thrown into the non-stop babycare, and dealing with terrible colic. Terrifyingly, at nine weeks of age, Olivia became feverish and floppy, and her parents rushed back to hospital. The baby had a virus and was given antibiotics and was soon fine, but it shattered Tina's and Tim's feelings yet again. They were interviewed when Olivia was six months old, and they were finally beginning to feel more relaxed. Tina wanted to give the advice to anyone with an ill baby, "not to think about the long-term future; treat every minute as precious."

Rosalyn's baby was thankfully fine, but the drama over her own health and a prolonged stay in a chaotic hospital were upsetting. "My high blood pressure wouldn't come down, and I was told to look out for spots in front of my eyes, which might herald the onset of a convulsion, heart attack or stroke. This was scary in itself, and I held my beautiful baby and wondered what her life would be like if I were to die. I became dreamy and found I couldn't speak or hear things properly. A blood test showed me to be dangerously anaemic, and I was given four pints of blood in an overnight transfusion. It wasn't painful, but I was traumatised by the whole experience for a long time afterwards."

When You Have to Find a Way Through Trauma

Congenital Conditions

Around 4% of babies are born with unusual conditions that are part of their congenital makeup. That's nearly 1 in 20 – quite a lot – so it might be concluded that abnormalities are in fact a normal feature of human life. Such conditions do not necessarily mean ill health, but they are usually regarded as handicaps, or having the potential for problems later in life. Cleft palate, strawberry marks, hole-in-the-heart and Down's syndrome are some of the better-known congenital conditions (bluntly called "birth defects").

Few parents would not experience some kind of trauma upon discovering that their baby has a congenital condition. It is in the very nature of parenting to be concerned about the health, happiness and future of your child. When the condition manifests itself in the very appearance of your baby, you may feel doubly horrified. Some conditions can be altered with surgery. If the operation takes place within days of birth then you are further traumatised by seeing your helpless newborn subjected to the degradation and discomfort of surgery. Then again, if surgery cannot be performed right away, you have the agony of waiting.

Conditions for which surgery has no answers are probably what parents dread the most and take longest to adjust to. A common, if not universal, fear during pregnancy is that you couldn't bear to have a handicapped child – that you couldn't bond or live with such a child. But it seems that all of us (or very, very nearly all of us) do eventually bond with our children, deeply so, even in the face of any initial feelings of shock and perhaps revulsion. Who knows – you may even come to love your child all the more because of the massive emotions that you experience in the process of coming to terms with a congenital condition.

Ian and Janine have a son, Ben, who has Down's Syndrome. Ian says: "We were offered the nuchal fold test at the first scan, which showed the possibility of Down's. We then had an amniocentesis, which confirmed that the baby, a boy, had it. Otherwise we wouldn't have thought about testing, because Janine was 26 at the time, not in an age risk bracket.

There was the ordeal of "should we abort", but we didn't. Surfing the Internet and dropping in at the cyber chatrooms of people round the world with this condition helped us come to that decision. For the rest of the pregnancy we learned all about the condition and various problems associated. I wouldn't say that we totally came to terms with it. We were probably as mentally prepared as we could be, but it was still a shock when he arrived, to see him for real and so obviously a Down's baby. He also had heart problems. It was a triple trauma – finding out about it, seeing it for real and then having the worry of operations. Family and friends were supportive, but there was a knife in the heart every time

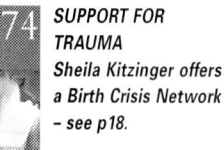

SUPPORT FOR TRAUMA
Sheila Kitzinger offers a Birth Crisis Network – see p18.

Your doctors or midwives might be able to recommend a support group for a particular type of congenital condition. The Internet is an excellent resource for every kind of disease – type in the name of the condition into a search engine.

In the worst-case scenario, it might help to contact the Stillbirth and Neonatal Death Society (SANDS) 28 Portland Place London W1N 4DE (020) 7436 5881

someone saw him for the first time, to see the smiles fade away or get falsely bigger. I think we got used to the way he looks in a couple of weeks, but it took a few months to stop worrying about other people's reactions. Or maybe it still hurts a little bit. In the meantime, Ben is now 11 months old and isn't self-conscious and forces everyone who knows him to love him back."

Gemma's son, Liam, has the rare condition achondroplasia (dwarfism), caused by a random genetic mutation: "We were warned that he might have the condition following a scan that showed unusual body dimensions, but we convinced ourselves it wasn't true. He looked so normal when he was born that we couldn't believe he had achondroplasia, but it was confirmed that he did.

I think we dealt with it quite well. Neither of us got depressed, but for weeks afterwards I did have odd moments or whole afternoons of feeling upset. I spent hours looking for evidence that he didn't have the condition, and that was probably the worst thing. Once I accepted that he truly did, it was much easier to move on and feel better about everything. Also, the lack of information about the condition didn't help, but once we learned more, we realised that it wasn't as bad as we had thought, and our doctors assured us that he would lead a fairly normal life. Liam himself makes it ok. Nine months later a lot of the pain has gone. It now feels like a dull ache that becomes apparent sometimes." (Gemma's stories about bonding are on pp203–204 and 212–213.)

BORN TOO SOON

Premature babies (by definition, those born before 37 weeks) often have health problems, and having an abrupt early end to pregnancy can be trauma in itself.

Christine had a routine check at 31 weeks, which showed an abnormally low level of amniotic fluid. After another 24 hours of tests, she had a caesarian. Her son, Ewan, needed help with breathing and feeding, and lived in an incubator for the first month: "From the moment the check showed those readings to now (ten weeks later) has been trauma, trauma, trauma. Both Ewan and I were dodgy for weeks on end. Everyone grumbles about NHS hospitals, but they were brilliant with us. We finally brought him home three weeks ago, but he is still tiny and looking after him is exhausting. I feel cheated on missing out on the last two months of pregnancy. Everyone says, at least I missed out on the stretch marks, but I had never sat down and thought about becoming a mother. A friend from my antenatal class is still waiting to have hers. I've abandoned my plan to return to work at four months." Like Tina, Christine had a powerful sense that these were the most important days of her life, and that nothing else must be allowed to distract her from her child.

PHASES IN COMING TO TERMS WITH TRAUMA

1. Shock/denial in the immediate aftermath.

2. Anger as the reality of the trauma sinks in. In the case of a birth trauma, it might be directed at medical professionals, or perhaps even God.

3. Self-blame – somehow it was all your own fault.

4. Depression – mood swings, apathy, disinterest in the world.

5. Acceptance – you rebuild life and the memories fade or do not hurt so much.

Such phases have been defined by psychologists and might be referred to if you seek help through counselling. Post-traumatic stress disorder can occur if such phases do not naturally progress.

BABYCARE CONTEXTS

77

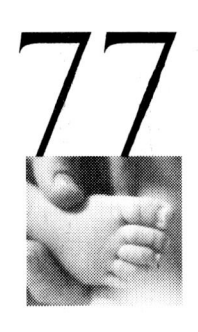

Contents

78 The Basics of Babycare

80 The Babycare Gurus

84 Contentious Issues

92 A Crying Checklist

100 Comforts for the Newborn

102 Typical Patterns of Baby Behaviour

The Basics of Babycare

*S*ome parts of babycare might be learnt from books, but the real learning comes from hands-on experience. This chapter looks at some of the contexts in babycare: a summary of tasks; what the experts say, and why they all contradict each other; routines; a collection of ideas about crying and comforts; and the typical changing patterns of behaviour through the first year.

The Everyday Tasks

The everyday tasks, as covered by the babycare manuals, are primarily about nourishment, hygiene and health. The amount of time attending to the first of these is a surprise to the majority of new parents. Newborn babies have very small stomachs. Therefore, expect to feed about every two to four hours in the first few weeks, while in between feeds your baby will be doing a mixture of sleeping, crying and sometimes showing an interest in the surroundings. Effectively, you will be living a 24-hour day. As the baby's stomach capacity grows and his sleep cycles mature, a pattern usually begins to develop that you can encourage into a more predictable 24-hour rhythm. Later in this book are two big chapters on Feeding and Sleeping.

Feeds precipitate excretion, which takes you into the realm of nappies. (You'll learn how to change a nappy the first time you do it.) First-time parents might wonder how often they should change a nappy. Basically, you ought to change a poo-filled nappy as soon as possible each time, but you won't know about every piddle. If you aim to change the nappy every three or four hours, you'll probably find several piddles' worth in them (to have a completely dry nappy after this time might be a sign of dehydration). Don't wake up your baby just to change a nappy, though, unless the nappy is very dirty. There's more about the changing patterns of digestion and excretion on pp102–109.

The more fun part of hygiene is bathing the baby. In the first few weeks this need only be once every few days, more of a sponge wash. (A full-on bath might be a slippery, frightening affair for both your newborn and you.) Within a couple of months, however, bathtime might be a fun way to end each day, whether a wash is needed or not.

Another obvious task is to stop the baby from coming to harm. In the earliest days, when the baby is helpless, unable to lift the weight of his own head, hazards come in such forms as over-heating or being sat on (by pets and other children for instance). Don't get into the habit of leaving your newborn lying on a changing table or adult bed, because within a few weeks will come the first shimmy to the side. Then there will be growing dexterity with objects (all of which go into the mouth), then rolling, sitting up, crawling and – very possibly within the space of 12 months – standing and walking. Each breakthrough can happen overnight, opening up the possibility of more and more hazards everywhere you go. A sort of inverse development takes place as the months go by – as the baby settles into a pattern of sleeping and feeding (thus giving you more time to yourself), so the baby's potential for coming to harm increases (thus increasing your need to be vigilant). Essentially, a child needs close attendance for several years. Thus, sharing responsibility is vital.

Building a Relationship

Pretty much everything else to do with babycare relates to your growing relationship together. With sleeping and feeding taking up the majority of time in the early weeks, initially there is little opportunity for much else. Touch and sound are probably the most useful senses to work with for communication at the beginning. But soon your baby's awareness of people and objects, and ability to engage with them will develop. The ways in which you can communicate and play with your child will broaden with every week that passes.

Beyond the basics, the best way to go about babycare is to slow down and simply respond to your baby. A huge amount of communication is non-verbal, and so you will almost certainly begin to understand the nature of your child quite rapidly. Engage in this conversation with eye contact, touch, sounds, expressions and words, but also take time to sit back and just watch your baby as he or she starts to take in the surrounding world. If you don't know your neighbourhood like the back of your hand already, this will be the time when you become familiar with every road and shop and inch of the nearest park.

The cornerstone of parenting is building a sense of security and happiness. The ways in which you encourage and foster independence while also nurturing deep and lifelong emotional bonds is the real substance of parenthood. And this is something that no babycare manual can ever give you the method for in a step-by-step fashion. Your own sense of security, possessiveness and satisfaction with parenting will change as the months go by, shaping your family dynamics. The ratio of time you need for yourself also has a bearing. Such dynamics are explored more in the chapter on Love and Triumph.

The Babycare Gurus

The first babycare manuals were published in the 19th century, and there has been a long stream of doctors and other professionals trying to influence practices in child-rearing. Every few decades sees a sea-change in attitudes as gurus come and go.

A Pint-Size History of Babycare

Infant mortality was high right up until the 20th century, not only from disease and bad sanitation but also from neglect and cruelty. For centuries, children appear to have been regarded – in Northern Europe at least – as inherently bad, and frequently beaten "for their own good". Wealthy families sent their newborn babies to wet nurses, and many didn't see their children for years.

Some social historians pinpoint Jean-Jacques Rousseau as the person who changed the perception of childhood. Through his book *Émile*, written in 1762, he called upon mothers not to send their babies away to be wet-nursed, and for children to be treated with more kindness. Along with the spread of other humanitarian ideas, children slowly started to get a better deal. Toys and children's books began to proliferate towards the end of the 18th century. William Buchan, a Yorkshireman and supporter of Rousseau, published books such as *Offices and Duties of Mothers* and *Advice to Mothers* around this time. In the Victorian era, Mrs Beeton became perhaps the first woman to give advice about feeding babies in her famous books on domestic science. Otherwise, the vast majority of babycare manuals were written by men, right up until the 1970s. These people helped shape the way the previous generations and our own were brought up.

Frederic Truby King (1858–1938) This was the famous doctor who decided that strict four-hour feeding and sleeping schedules were ideal and that playing and cuddles should be strictly limited. A baby should always be left to cry so as not to be spoilt. His ideas were very influential on our grandparents' generation, though widely condemned now. The four-hour feeding policy was followed slavishly in maternity hospitals right up to the 1970s. In his favour, however, his focus on the importance of nutrition (including breastfeeding) drastically reduced infant mortality in the first half of the 20th century.

Edward Bowlby and Donald Winnicott These two threw out some of King's ideas and influenced 1950s ideals about mother-baby attachment. Winnicott famously declared that there is no such thing as a baby, only a mother-baby unit. (A father had little role other than as disciplinarian.) Working mothers were villified, and nursery places were reduced for a few decades.

Dr Benjamin Spock (1903–1998) This American doctor became the most influential babycare guru of all time. His *Common Sense Book of Baby and Child Care*, first written in 1946, went on to sell 50 million copies around the world (only the Bible has sold more). In his view, children should pretty much be allowed to do whatever they want in their own time. People who didn't like his ideas blamed him for the permissive, "anything goes" society of the 60s and 70s. Like virtually all the other male childcare theorists, he firmly believed that mothers should do most of the donkey work of parenting. Otherwise, he was relatively lenient on mothers – telling them they didn't have to breastfeed if they didn't want, and that they, not the doctors, were the real experts about their own children. Your own parents might have brought you up on Dr Spock.

BABYCARE GURUS TODAY

Revised editions of Dr Spock's books are still available, but other gurus have also emerged since the 1970s. Most have taken on and adapted Dr Spock's "child-centred" approach. But some disagree with this approach and give advice for "adult-led" parenting (see also the Controversial Issues section that follows this). Only a few tread the middle ground. This list of the most popular babycare experts today is alphabetical.

Robin Barker She is Australia's best-selling babycare writer, though relatively unknown elsewhere, offering advice built up from 30 years' experience as a midwife, health visitor and mother. The 600-page *Baby Love* volume is divided into age-band chapters up to one year, offering various ideas to help if the going gets rough with crying, breastfeeding and sleeplessness. Because of her "middle-of-the-road" approach, she was invited to be one of the contributors to this book. Her summary of the changing patterns of baby behaviour starts on p102, and her view on breastfeeding is on p132.

Steve Biddulph Another Australian, Steve Biddulph has written a number of popular books on parenting, including *Raising Boys* and *The Secret of Happy Children*. His style is a mix of practical suggestions and light-hearted asides, very much written from hands-on experience.

The Babycare Gurus

Dr Richard Ferber He's not a babycare guru as such, but worth mentioning as one of the world's leading authorities on sleep in babies and children. Countless tired parents have turned to his book, *Solve Your Child's Sleep Problems*, after months of broken nights. The book covers sleep disorders in babies over six months or so – broken night sleep, nightmares, night terrors, sleepwalking and bed-wetting in older children. His advice has been the door to heaven for countless parents, but some people have criticised his sleep training methods for being like a "baby boot camp".

Gina Ford With her phenomenally successful *The Contented Little Baby Book* (1998), maternity nurse Gina Ford gives pretty much the total opposite advice to the child-centred gurus. Out goes demand feeding and waiting for a sleep pattern to develop. In comes a structured day in which every sleep, feed and burping session are timed to the minute. Her slim book gives a changing routine from the age of two weeks to a year. There is no doubt that her routines can work for some (take a look at the hundreds of rave reviews on www.amazon.com). But many people also find her no-nonsense, opinionated tone too much to stomach. Interestingly, a number of her supporters say that they have adapted her routine to suit, despite the fact that Gina Ford is adamant that the timings she gives have to be strict for the routine to work. See also pp86, 87, 89 and 172.

Christopher Green Yet another Australian, here is a consultant paediatrician with a humorous outlook on the tough world of babies and young children. Consult his *Babies*, *Toddler Taming* and *Beyond Toddlerdom* to see what you are in for over the next decade. His common-sense advice is popular with parents finding life with their beloved youngsters a bit of a strain.

Tracy Hogg *Secrets of the Baby Whisperer* has a range of tips from a Yorkshire-born nanny who practices in the States. Another one who doesn't like the philosophy of demand feeding, she emphasises the importance of interpreting cues from babies. A central part of her approach is a loose, three-hour recurring routine that she gives the acronym EASY (eating, activity, sleep and you). She also divides babies into temperament types.

Penelope Leach The most influential guru since Dr Spock, this British psychologist and mother started writing childcare manuals in the 1970s. Titles such as *Your Baby and Child*, *Babyhood* and *Children First* are still going strong, having sold millions around the world. Her basic child-centred philosophy is to follow

---

WEBSITES FOR PARENTS
There are hundreds of parenting websites, especially American-based ones, such as www.parentsoup.com. Many are online magazines, with features, chat rooms, "ask an expert" forums, product reviews and online shopping facilities.

Some of the better British-based websites:
- www.parentalk.co.uk
- www.b4baby.com
- www.mumsnet.com

the baby's lead always, and that you can never spoil a child with too much attention. She has a vast following of mothers. However, she has also been heavily attacked for building an idealistic vision of motherhood that is perhaps impossible to achieve. For example, she suggests that one of the main ways to demonstrate your love is to answer every cry promptly. Many parents find that this isn't always practical or desirable, especially when sleep training, but their love is not necessarily diminished by this.

William Sears One of the most controversial gurus in the States for his theories about "attachment parenting", which include co-sleeping (see p91 and p163). If you are interested, browse his website, www.askdrsears.com.

Miriam Stoppard *Conception, Pregnancy and Birth* is the UK's most popular baby title, and Dr Stoppard has long been considered a leading authority on babycare and family life. Well illustrated and easy to read, her books are among the few with advice for fathers, too. Some parents have suggested that the information is too broad brush to be of much use when faced with the realities of birth and the early postnatal period. But two women interviewed for this book found her advice reassuring and a good reference source.

Childcare Authority Sources

The What to Expect Series Written by Arlene Eisenberg, Heidi E. Murkoff and Sandee E. Hathaway, *What to Expect: the First Year* is a weighty tome that has been phenomenally popular in the States since 1989 and, perhaps surprisingly given its pervasive American slant, has also sold well in Britain. The main sections cover each month of development, with a lot of content in the form of answers to parents' questions. There's advice about everything from "black stool" to questions of "is my baby gifted?" and ways of "easing back into sex". It is astonishingly detailed, the most comprehensive modern babycare manual. The advice given is with great deference to the American Academy of Pediatrics, which is good if you want an official methodology, but not so good if you dislike a conservative, patrician style.

The Birth to Five Manual The UK's health authority manual, given free to every new mother, is the British parent's first port of call to find the latest official information on everything relating to postnatal health. It is very good on weaning and childhood illnesses. Written by health committee for the whole social spectrum, it does not attempt to enter the fray on the more culturally charged aspects of babycare, such as bed-sharing and routines.

OTHER MANUALS WRITTEN BY COMMITTEES
• *The Great Ormond Street New Baby and Child Care Book (1997)*

• *The NCT Complete Book of Baby Care (1999)*

BOOKS ABOUT SOCIAL ISSUES
• *The Myth of Motherhood* by Aminatta Forna – how society has shaped the notion of motherhood in Western culture.

• *Baby Wisdom* by Deborah Jackson – looks at practices in other cultures, often comparing our own unfavourably (see p91).

• *Misconceptions* by Naomi Wolf – all the hidden difficulties new mothers face.

• *The Parent Trap* by Maureen Freely – how the media creates parenting ideals.

Contentious Issues

Much to do with parenting is subject to conflicting opinions, contradictory advice and differing moral agendas. What the health authority says, what the books say, and what your own mother and friends say might all be different, and you will have to decide things for yourself. Here are the main issues.

Feeding Issues

Breastfeeding is the most discussed element of babycare. Currently being promoted out of its near-redundancy during our own mothers' generation, it's the subject of classes offered by the NHS, NCT and pro-breastfeeding organisations. Indeed, it is about the only aspect of babycare that antenatal classes cover. And whole books are written on the subject, for while it may appear to be the most natural practice on Earth, breastfeeding is also associated with numerous physical and emotional problems and social issues. A close look at the workings, benefits and politics of breastfeeding is on pp112–151.

The average age for beginning the process of weaning onto "solids" has changed over the years, generally getting later. The official recommended age to start weaning is now four to six months. This is because studies have shown that babies' digestive systems cannot adequately cope with anything other than milk (preferably human milk) before the age of four months. Any advice you might hear to start weaning onto solids earlier than four months might come from an older generation (your grandmother, perhaps) who did not know there was anything wrong with weaning at three months or even earlier. Leaving it later than six months is also regarded as a problem, when nutritive elements from other foods start to become important for optimum health.

Sleep Issues

Hot on the heels of feeding come questions about where babies should sleep, how much sleep they need, and how they might be encouraged to "sleep through" the night. The babycare gurus and manuals all have different approaches to these topics: some contradict each other, while others keep out of the fray by barely covering the topic of sleep at all. Sleep issues and up-to-date advice about how to minimize the risk of cot death are on pp153–197.

COLIC AND TEETHING

Colic is still the old chestnut of "nobody really knows what causes it and some say it doesn't exist at all". Babycare advisers, from doctors to colic drop manufacturers, peddle various theories and sympathy. The only thing you can safely comfort yourself with if your baby seems to have it is that it's not a serious condition, just a miserable one involving an awful lot of crying. For more on the subject see p95.

Teething is a bit different. Possibly the majority of parents believe that teething can cause grumpiness, pain, sleeplessness, even stomach upsets, fever and a host of other things. But it may surprise parents to know that the majority of babycare experts either categorically state that the emergence of teeth doesn't cause any of these things, or at least play down the idea that teething causes problems. *Birth to Five* doesn't suggest that teeth cause problems, but acknowledges that many parents say that they do. See p98.

ROUTINES

Routines are extremely contentious. In babycare literature are two main lines of thought. On the one hand, there are some babycare gurus – probably a minority at the moment – who recommend a daily routine for feeding, sleeping and activities from birth, saying that this can be practically and emotionally beneficial for both mother and child. Opposing them is the child-centred camp (e.g. Penelope Leach, Miriam Stoppard and the NCT) who give the impression that routines are cruel for young babies and can sabotage both breastfeeding and bonding.

What is the new parent to make of this major rift in advice? It helps to understand the history of the argument, which relates to the swing in popular babycare practice during the 20th century. In the first half of the 20th century the childcare doctor Truby King (see p80) recommended a routine for babies from birth, timed to the minute, which included four-hourly feeds during the day, no night feeding, little physical contact and recommendations that babies should be left to cry, even when hungry and out in the cold, so as not to "spoil" the child. In essence, it was a regime of near-military harshness, yet his advice was highly influential in various parts of the Western world for several decades. Many of our grandparents would have been brought up like this.

But with the advent of the permissive 1960s, Benjamin Spock's advice to do the complete opposite – just let babies and children do what they want in their own time – meant that "routine" became a demonised concept in many parenting circles. Childhood memories of strict timetables and a tragic lack of physical affection may have been cause for our parents' generation to rebel. In this way, the idea of routines became a polemical issue – for or against.

Contentious Issues

For the past couple of decades, most of the popular babycare writers have been "child-centred", saying that you should let your baby lead the way from birth and eventually he will fall into his own pattern for feeding, sleeping and so on. There's no definitive age by which this is guaranteed to happen – every baby is different. (See also Robin Barker's view on p107.) The *Birth to Five* book, oracle of the Health Authority, skirts around the issue ("routine" does not even appear in its index). The controversy about routines is also tied up with issues about "feeding on demand" (see p134), attachment theories (see p91) and sleep politics (see p162). Generally speaking, pro-breastfeeding campaigners and family-bed supporters don't like routines.

Of the babycare gurus who do advocate a routine these days, thankfully they do not suggest one that is so harsh as Truby King's. Gina Ford (see p82) has become today's best-known guru to fervently promote the benefits of a strict routine. Health professionals that you will come into contact with – midwives, paediatricians and health visitors – are also bound to have different opinions about routines.

One aim of this book, however, is to point out that there is a very large middle-ground barely covered in modern babycare literature (either because the experts come from one or the other camp, or because the middle-ground is harder to define or give instructions for). Many parents know, through trial and error, that as the weeks and months go by you can develop a rough routine that is partly baby-led and partly parent-led. All the parents of older babies interviewed for this book had some kind of daily routine going within one to six months of birth.

Developing a part baby-led, part parent-led routine arises out of observing and responding to your child's unique needs and personality while also coaxing habits into a pattern that allows the family household to function smoothly and happily from day to day. In some families, the daily routine, or parts of it, are adhered to more strictly than in others. The parents become experts about the minutiae of their own child's daily rhythm.

At the very least, whether they think of it as a routine or not, the vast majority of parents like to instigate a difference between day and night, to help the baby get used to night as the time for the longest sleep. According to sleep researchers, newborn babies do not have circadian rhythms (see p161), but by about six months they do. It is impossible for a baby to fall into a circadian rhythm without some form of intervention from the parent, even if that is merely being put to bed at roughly the same time each evening.

Many parents describe a sense of relief, a growing feeling of stability and more confidence in their parenting skills, once the baby starts to settle into a routine. In fact, the issue of routines is really only controversial with regard to very young babies. Most people will agree that older babies and children thrive

---

THE CHILD-CENTRED APPROACH
The "child-centred" approach prevails in most modern baby-care manuals and formal teachings. With this, you learn how to fulfil your child's needs, generally by following the child's lead.

In the editor's opinion, this approach is flawed because it overlooks the intense symbiotic relationship between parent and child, and the dynamics of the family as a whole. Aspects such as adult needs and desires, fears, possessiveness and the altered sense of self as a parent are barely acknowledged. A better approach is to look at the changing needs of the family.

emotionally within the familiarity and stability of a daily routine. The world isn't such an unquantifiable, confusing and terrifying place to a toddler if he knows roughly what is going to happen next. It's the degree to which the parent can or should instigate the routine that is contentious.

Routines at any age don't necessarily have to be strict, although some parents swear by strict timing. Basically, you'll get to know what leeway is in whatever routine develops, and you'll probably find that the routine changes in phases as your child's physical and mental capacities develop.

Parents' Views about Routines

There was a huge response from parents who were asked for their views on the subject of routines, and what kind of routine had developed for them as the months went by. (Their babies were all more than three months old.) A range of contrasting views and anecdotes are included here.

Alice: "I read somewhere that the mother and baby should be regarded as a single unit, that is, their activities and behaviour must suit both of them to some degree. Therefore, the balance can't totally be in favour of the baby, or of the mother. But, having said that, I believe that at the beginning, you do have to be led by the baby. Trying to enforce strict meal times to a newborn is cruel and ridiculous, both to the baby and yourself. However, as time goes on, the baby's behaviour can begin to be led by you. I found that my baby became clearly more able to cope with different things as he grew older. So, at five months, I felt it was okay to let him cry himself to sleep when he was tired but resisting taking a nap. This measure was necessary in order to establish some kind of daytime routine that a childminder could take over, when I went back to work. Yet, at five weeks, I think it would have been cruel to do this – both to the baby and to me.

I was quite influenced by Gina Ford about a month after the birth but now I regard her book as a gimic, even if it does have some good bits of advice and information sprinkled through it. I cannot imagine anyone really following her advice on routines and thereby totally sacrificing their own life."

Amy dislikes the notion of rigid routines, whatever the age of the child. "My view is that all babies are different – some might be happy to go into a routine, but others aren't and shouldn't be forced to. I think that parents are hung up on routines in this country. We are so obsessed with clock-watching, but there's a more natural pace of life in a lot of other countries, where it simply doesn't matter if the children are still running around at midnight or want to spend two hours snacking or picking at dinner. Soon after the birth of my first child, I realised that you have to slow down, live life at the child's level and speed. Trying to impose a feeding and sleep schedule is a waste of effort and sanity."

Georgina, a mother of twins: "Partly because of my mum's influence, and partly because I have two babies, I have been very "unfashionable" in the way I have looked after Sam and Eva these first 12 weeks. I have opted for a very strict routine and stuck to it. Both babies have got into quite a good pattern and feed and settle well. I would recommend a routine to anyone -- especially for mums with more than one child to look after. It means you know where you are, the babies become familiar with the routine and it is easier to get people to help as you know what's happening when. I am also strict about bath times and bed times too -- from my limited experience Sam and Eva seem happier that way.

While timings are strict, we're not totally tied by routine. They sleep on sheepskins rather than a bed, which means I can take them anywhere and put them down to sleep – on someone else's floor, in a borrowed pram, on the grass under a tree... It makes life with babies much more flexible and means you don't have to take loads of kit everywhere."

Jacqui: "I remember my NCT teacher being scathing about routines – "a routine for the baby is a routine for you too". She presented it like not having a routine would mean freedom. I can now see what she means, but personally have found a routine much easier to live with. Not having a routine in the beginning meant that I could take Chloë in a sling to go shopping and to restaurants with my friends – she could sleep and feed whenever she wanted. But that stage only lasted about two months. Now I never go to a restaurant because she wants to crawl around, and if she's tired she won't just sit in her pushchair and sleep. She grouches until we get home and I put her in the cot for a nap. So she has forced me into a routine, not the other way round."

Ruth: "I'd read Penelope Leach and consulted friends (my parents can't remember much). I was ready to feed on demand, but equally I was keen to establish a night-time sleeping routine just for my own sanity. Being a big baby, she slept for four hours at night without needing food, and at four months just slept through for 12 hours. I was fairly relaxed about daytime feeding and sleeping, the only thing I was rigid about (and still am seven months on) is bedtime – a bath, milk, bed routine which I started doing within the first 10 days. It took some weeks to get established, and until four or five months she occasionally cried when I left the room. I wouldn't leave her crying but just kept feeding her and putting her back to bed. She now goes to bed without complaint.

I have read Gina Ford's book – with incredulity – I'm sure her routines work, but it leaves no time for adult life."

Annette: "In the first month, we tended to keep Annie with us and let her sleep whilst we were downstairs in the living room and then all go up together. We did this partly as she was feeding quite often and also we wanted to have her near us. We do now (at three months) have a bedtime routine in which Annie will have a bath at about 6–6.30pm, a feed at about 6.45 and then upstairs to bed. She will then have another feed at about 10.30–11pm and generally sleeps through until 6.30 or 7am. She will have two, sometimes three naps per day. However, these are not as structured as the evening routine, and a lot depends on what we are doing during the day."

Stella: "I think everyone has a different idea about what "routine" means. The image conjured up when you first hear about a routine for a baby is Nanny in a starched collar saying "no fussing, time for Baby's bath!" My two children and I have a loose routine which either they or I am allowed to break at least three times a week. Some friends are so obsessed with their routine that they miss the baby massage class because it clashes with nap time. Then I've got another friend who says her son doesn't want to or need to sleep in the day. Yet he is always grumpy or "teething", in the way that mine are if they are tired, and I think why doesn't she try harder to make him take a daytime nap?"

Eve is fervently in favour of routines, and had a lot to say on the subject: "My mum and dad were Seventies hippies and brought up my brother and me on Dr Spock – routine was a dirty word. But now that I have eight months' experience of motherhood behind me, I am totally in favour of routines – sorry mum, but I guess it's true that we're a more uptight generation than yours. Harry spent the first month either feeding or crying or falling asleep on top of me so that I had no time off from him at all, not even to clean my teeth. It was like we were just dragging ourselves through endless days. He was a terrible baby, and I was a terrible mother.

Some friends have an older baby who was very settled from a young age, and at about five weeks I decided to apply her routine to Harry. I started putting him in his basket to sleep rather than always wait for him to fall asleep on the nipple, to put him to nap three times a day and to bed for the night at 7.30pm, then not take him out of the bedroom until the next morning, and to make sure he breastfed every two or three hours between 7.30am and 7.30pm, which sometimes meant waking him up from a long nap. I also made sure he had three

SLEEP ROUTINES
Helping to establish a good 24-hour sleep pattern over the course of the first six months or so can be the defining factor in a routine. Ideas on how to do this are covered in the Sleep chapter. All other elements of the day and night – the baby's feeds, activity and play, and your own adult life – can fall into place around a rough sleep routine. (That's the editor's view, anyway.)

set playtimes during the day, once under the baby gym and the others with me chatting to him and showing him contrasty objects. I'm telling you that within three days there was a definite difference – less crying overall, and within a few weeks he was in a fairly predictable routine. I say "fairly" because he was still waking at least once in the night, often between 3am and 5am, and sometimes he was difficult to settle during the day. But this was comparatively easy to cope with, and I started enjoying motherhood at that stage. I was still fully breastfeeding as well. We realised that it was very important to structure the rest of our lives around the routine. He falls asleep quite easily in the car, so we started timing car journeys to coincide with a nap time. Also, we were at a party one evening, but he got tired – we left rather than trying to rock him to sleep with all the noise going on.

I think it was at three-and-a-half months that we found we didn't have to follow the exact same routine as our friend's baby, and not have to be too strict. Since six months we have had a fantastic time – a day with five minutes of crying is unusual (sometimes at bedtime), he sleeps for nearly 11 hours at night, and I have so much more energy. It's good to have the evening to yourselves: to talk, watch telly in peace, read a book, make love even."

Sarah: "Tilly got into a sort of routine at about four months, which was a relief. Since she got into the routine I've been quite careful to keep her sleeps on track each day because I have found that the tireder she becomes, the harder she finds it to sleep. I put her to bed whether she looks tired or not. Usually I go back ten minutes later and she has fallen asleep. It was when we went on holiday and had to break the routine that we realised how important it is to her. Every time there's some disruption to her routine, she's unsettled and cries a lot. It's her routine, not ours, by the way: we always adapt our own lives to fit in with hers."

Valerie: "I didn't know there was any controversy about routines – maybe because I've never read any books, just followed the way my sisters have raised their children. Some babies seem to be born in a routine, and others need to be coaxed into one as soon as possible, for their own sake and yours."

ATTACHMENT VERSUS INDEPENDENCE

The way a parent relates to a child is always a concurrent mix of encouraging attachment and independence. This duality begins at birth and is forever more in a state of flux: the child comes out and breathes independently while you fulfil her every other need. Within a few months you are enjoying her reciprocal affections while also relieved that she is trying to sit up, eat finger foods – her

Babycare Contexts

dependence on you is slightly less. A few more months and she is running around, sometimes craving comfort, other times annoyed when you assert authority. Eventually she will leave home, hopefully with a lifelong sense of security that you have fostered over the years. But your relief at her independence is perhaps tempered with nostalgia for the closeness of the early days.

The relationship of attachment and independence is an essential part of each family's dynamic and would not be contentious at all but for the fact that it can be influenced by social attitudes. For instance, babies brought up on the methodology of Truby King were pushed towards independence much faster than babies brought up on Penelope Leach (see pp80–83).

It has often been observed that the Western world places great emphasis on independence and the individual, whereas many other cultures create more attachments within the social group – the nuclear family versus the extended family. Some people say that we encourage independence too soon in our culture – making a baby sleep in a different bed, for instance, when she would be happier to sleep in our arms. There is a body of childcare literature, starting with Jean Liedloff's *The Continuum Concept* in the Seventies and continuing through to the Nineties with William Sears' *The Baby Book*, Katie Allison Granju's *Attachment Parenting* and Deborah Jackson's *Three in a Bed* and *Baby Wisdom*, which looks to other cultures for inspiration, with ideas about "natural" bonding, including breastfeeding on demand to fulfill all comfort sucking, co-sleeping and carrying in a sling rather than having a pram. Like the drive to encourage breastfeeding, it can be a proselytising ideology. Parents tend to end up either for it or against it, rarely indifferent.

SMACKING

Finally, you might be justifiably surprised to see the contentious topic of smacking in a book about the first year of parenthood. Many people think of it as something that relates to the toddler years and beyond (whether they are for or against it). But NSPCC research in 2001 concluded that many British children under 12 months are regularly hit, with more than half being smacked at least weekly – an almost unbelievable figure. In this context, smacking cannot possibly be regarded as an issue about discipline – babies cannot foresee the consequences of their actions. It is a sign of uncontrolled rage and aggression in the adult and potentially dangerous, as shown by the statistic that a baby under 12 months is five times more likely than an older child to be killed by a carer. The exhausted parent who is cracking under the stress of living with a baby needs practical and emotional support, not the tacit approval of the pro-smacking lobby. A crying checklist for harrassed parents follows...

POTTY TRAINING
Whereas the Truby King generations started potty training at nine months, we now leave it much later. The modern concensus of advice is to wait for the child to start showing signs of wanting to use a potty (such as being aware of wanting to pee and being distressed by a dirty nappy). This could begin to happen as early as 18 months or not until three years.

In some countries, especially hot ones, in which nappy rash can be more of a problem, or nappies aren't used at all, there is a greater drive towards toilet training than in our society.

Potty training is something a lot of parents become competitive about, but whatever age you start the process, take it very gently.

A Crying Checklist

Trying to quell the crying directs much of what we do at first with a new baby. A sense of satisfaction springs from the ability to soothe the cries of a child. But often in the early weeks (and sporadically thereafter), there will be times when we have difficulty soothing those cries, despite all our efforts.

> **EARLY DYNAMICS**
> Responding to your child's crying forms one of the first dynamics in your relationship with each other.
> The child cries, you let her feed and the crying ceases. Later the cry returns, and you attend to her once again. Slowly, you become familiar with your child, whilst at the same time you yourself change.

CRYING IN CONTEXT

In Victorian Britain and even up to our own mothers' generation (and slightly into our own), a widely held belief was that babies need to exercise their lungs through crying, and parking the child in a pram at the end of the garden to yell it out was the done thing. Nowadays, we are generally taught that babies always cry for a "legitimate" reason, such as hunger or discomfort – thus the onus is on you to find the reason. This more baby-friendly attitude is appealing in principle. Unfortunately, in practice the reasons for crying are often not clear. We leave the guiltless realm of believing that crying is a sign of good health, so the parent is left full of worry and feelings of inadequacy. Don't become despondent thinking that you are failing your baby if you do not always understand the crying. Also bear in mind that trivial reasons can sometimes result in an excessive amount of wailing.

Soothing your baby is likely to be a big preoccupation for you at first: trying to identify the cause each time; using comfort mechanisms (see pp100–101) if no cause can be found; and slowly learning how to anticipate and prevent the crying from starting; and even when it's ok to ignore it.

Sometimes crying really is inconsolable, and the affects of it on a tired parent can be profound. If the crying is "getting to you", leave your baby in a safe place in another room for a while (a quarter of an hour maybe) and seek emotional and practical support from family, friends, health visitors or anyone else sympathetic. The helpline CRY-SIS offers support (see p94). Definitely seek help if you find yourself perpetually resorting to leaving the baby to cry somewhere else: this could be a sign that you are suffering from nervous exhaustion or postnatal depression, both of which are eased with the help of other people to share the practicalities of babycare.

If you are in the first month or two of parenthood, be comforted by the sure and certain fact that the crying will decrease as the weeks go by, and your baby relaxes and learns to communicate in more refined ways. The crying may sound like abject misery in your baby, but it may stem from a minor reason. You are in the very worst of it; the crying will never be so unfathomable as it is now; the situation WILL improve; and you have the sympathies of every other parent who can remember what it was like at the beginning.

The "checklist" that follows is the editor's compilation of the kind of ideas about crying that are bandied around today. Some are controversial and subject to extreme views. Also consider that babies vary a lot in sensitivity, and that parents vary a lot in their own sensitivity to their babies' sensitivity…

HUNGER

Likely type of cry With a hungry newborn baby, the likely sign is a cry that becomes increasingly loud and insistent (but this is not to say that all loud and insistent crying is a sign of hunger).

Other possible signs A newborn baby's rooting reflex (p115) also indicates hunger – this reflex decreases after a couple of months.

What to do A few decades ago, when four-hour feeding schedules were broadly recommended, mothers were discouraged from feeding their babies in between the scheduled times even if the baby was crying and clearly hungry. This idea is largely discredited now. By contrast, mothers are now often advised to "feed on demand". In the early days following birth, midwives will probably encourage you to let your baby suckle whenever he cries – this is because frequent suckling is the only way that his tiny stomach can digest enough milk at this early stage and it helps to establish your milk supply.

"Feeding on demand" is looked at in more detail on pp134–137. Some experts argue that it is an over-simplified phrase that can be taken too literally. Not all crying means that your baby is demanding food, even though the offer of food and the distraction of sucking may comfort him. Snacking frequently rather than taking a smaller number of full feeds is not usually considered a problem for the baby; but as time goes by it may become a problem for you (see p138). If you always "plug in" rather than exploring other reasons for why your baby cries, then you might become exhausted from breastfeeding.

A baby's food and sleep requirements are closely linked and constantly changing, and understanding them can be the most difficult part of babycare. Rhythms for feeding and sleeping are covered on pp134–151 and 181–194. The genuine hunger cry will become less common once you can anticipate the baby's appetite and offer feeds before he starts to make the "demand".

EACH CHILD IS DIFFERENT
If you spend much time on an open postnatal ward, you will soon notice that not only does each newborn child look different, but the cries all sound distinctive too. The editor's baby went "wah-wah-wah", the one opposite went "grrrrrrr-oooo" and the rest of the ward was a mix of "yowowwayowow", "hurrerr-hurrer", "eea-wee-eea" etc etc.

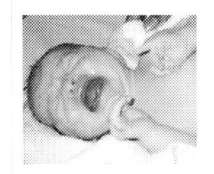

A Crying Checklist

TIREDNESS

Likely type of cry Irregular fussing that becomes increasingly forceful and may easily be mistaken for hunger or boredom.

Other possible signs Maybe yawning, squirming, arching the back, turning away from light. Once arm control has developed, rubbing at the eyes or thumb sucking is a possibility. Irritability and clumsiness, hyperactivity, bursts of energy but limited attention are common. Signs of tiredness might be difficult to identify in the newborn but are increasingly obvious as the baby gets older.

What to do Newborn babies often drift off to sleep of their own accord, usually after feeding or when in some rhythmic motion, such as in a car. They may often sleep with bright lights and loud noise around them, which older children and adults may not be able to do. However, it seems that even newborn babies may sometimes have difficulty going to sleep, particularly if they are excited by their surroundings, and they will cry from tiredness. It is widely accepted that as babies get older they can find it increasingly difficult to shut out the world and relax into sleep, and nap times and bedtime might become the main source of crying.

Experts vary in their opinions as to how long babies can stay awake before tiring, and how much sleep they need. If your baby is not yet in a recognisable rhythm or routine of sleeping and feeding, then tiredness may be difficult to identify. As a rough guide, however, if more than two-and-a-half or three hours have gone by since your newborn woke up (and she has fed well in that time), then it is worth considering that she may be crying from tiredness rather than hunger or colic or another discomfort. As with other types of crying, she may stop crying if you distract her attention with new stimuli, but the crying will come back with increasing forcefulness because her already tired body and mind are being over-stimulated and stressed. She may need to wind down from this state before she can sleep.

If you think your baby is crying from tiredness (and you have ruled out hunger, illness, discomfort etc), then you could try putting the baby in her bed in a quiet, darkened room for a while. Away from the constant stimulation her cries may become intermittent and then perhaps she will sleep.

As noted under hunger, feeding and sleeping are closely linked. A tired newborn baby can often be "fast-tracked" into sleep by being fed, even if she doesn't really need the food. However, feeding-to-sleep doesn't always work, it works less and less as the weeks go by, and, as noted under the hunger cry, a vast amount of feeding and comfort sucking may become exhausting for the breastfeeding mother. Swaddling, rocking and dummies are among other comforts (pp100–101). There is a lot more about sleep on pp153–197.

CRY-SIS HELPLINE
(020) 7404 5011
7 days a week,
8am –11pm.
This is a helpline for parents who perhaps feel close to breaking point with the stress of babycare. Lines are manned by other parents who understand the problems generated by excessive crying from a baby. They have been trained to offer reassurance and practical suggestions. You will be put in touch with someone in your area.

Wind

Likely type of cry Short-lived squeals.

Other possible signs Belching, farting, straining, squirming, going rigid and red in the face are all easy signs to identify in a baby with wind.

What to do Burping and breaking wind loudly are a normal part of the newborn infant's day, and he may also strain and cry while trying to excrete or pass wind through his newly functioning intestines. (Advice to change the nappy is usually on crying checklists, for obvious reasons, but anecdotal evidence suggests that it's mainly older children who are actually upset at wearing a dirty nappy.)

The practice of "burping" babies is popular in our culture – holding them upright and rubbing and patting their backs after a feed so that they burp up the air swallowed with the milk. Modern babycare writers vary in their enthusiasm for this practice. Some suggest that you should spend a few minutes after each feed to help your baby burp up every last bit of air; others point out that the practice does not exist in other cultures and that it is largely unnecessary because discomfort from wind is not that great. The amount of wind (and posset) should decrease after a couple of months as the baby's digestive system matures.

Colic

Likely type of cry Shrill, loud, persistent, inconsolable.

Other possible signs Often said to happen at the same time of day, usually in the evening, pulling legs up to stomach.

What to do Advice about colic is frustratingly contradictory because the term is used in so many different contexts. Some experts say that colic is not a separate condition at all, but a catch-all term for all kinds of unexplained crying. With this view, forceful crying that keeps occuring in the evening – along with any associated straining and twisting – can possibly be regarded as a symptom of over-tiredness and stress, not a problem with digestion at all.

Voicing a contrary opinion, the makers of colic drops and gripe water say that colic is a severe form of trapped wind, caused by tiny bubbles of air in the baby's intestine. The trapped wind can be treated with simethicone in colic drops, which joins the little bubbles together so that they form big bubbles that can be expelled more easily. In the manufacturers' marketing literature they talk about the signs of colic including pulling the knees up to the chest, and a rock-hard stomach, not necessarily in the evening.

Then again, a lot of people talk about colic as a pattern of crying in the late afternoon or evening. A number of theories are in vogue. One is that the

A Crying Checklist

mother's breastmilk is used up by mid-afternoon and so the baby is perpetually hungry in the evening. If you suspect that your breastmilk supply is insufficient see pp139–141 and seek support. Other theories are that too much foremilk (see p117) or over-feeding can lead to intestinal discomfort. But breastfeeding experts are not agreed on these ideas.

Foods eaten by the mother during the day such as orange juice and cabbage and spicy food have been blamed by some. The solution in these cases is to avoid various foods that might be causing digestive disturbances. You may be able to identify something quite easily. But before you go radically restricting your own diet, or blaming breastfeeding if it is otherwise working for you, bear in mind that "colic" is also reported in bottle-fed babies, and that theories like these are totally rubbished by some experts. Some bottle manufacturers claim that their products reduce colic, because they reduce the likelihood of air going down with the milk. But they don't claim to have eradicated colic in bottle-fed babies.

The bottom line is that "colic" is a term for any inconsolable crying, which all young babies seem to have here and there, some much more than others. The age at which "colic" can strike is also subject to different views – from birth, two weeks, three weeks etc. See Robin Barker's summary of the possible unsettled phase, p104. Most people agree that "colic" (whatever it is) ceases at about three months. One way or another, if your baby is inconsolable for hours and you cannot find the cause, it may give you some small, scant relief to be able to give the crying the name of "colic".

If your baby seems colicky, try the normal range of comforts (see pp100–101). Laying the colicky baby on his tummy, maybe over your knee, is popular. Massage is also claimed by some to help soothe colic. Baby massage classes are available in some areas – if you want to try it at home, use a liberal amount of almond or vegetable oil and warm your hands to stroke and massage the little body. If you've tried everything, just place your baby in bed to give yourself a break and maybe have your own cry too. Think this: your baby is relatively well if he can bawl his lungs out (a weak cry is the real sign of illness).

Too Hot

Likely type of cry Could be whimpering, intermittently or insistently crying (or, more dangerously, not crying at all).

Other possible signs Hot in the body and at the back of neck, perhaps sweaty and red, straining (or, more dangerously, not moving at all).

What to do These days there is more talk about the dangers of a baby becoming over-heated than too cold. (See Avoiding Cot Death, p196.) Babies can't regulate their body temperature very well. Too many layers or central heating that's turned up too high, including in the car, can be a danger area. Check the skin temperature on the body or back of the neck and take off layers etc. If over-heating was the problem then the baby will hopefully soon stop crying as he cools down.

Too Cold

Likely type of cry As with over-heating, could be whimpering, intermittently or insistently crying (or, more dangerously, not crying at all).
Other possible signs Paleness, or blue tinge to skin, bottom lip quivering, torso cool to touch – the limbs are often cooler than the body and so are not a reliable indicator – perhaps limp. Note that newborns cannot shiver.
What to do Minimise the time spent in a cold environment. A newborn baby might cry at the feel of cool air on her naked skin, such as when being changed. She will probably soon stop crying when clothed again. This does not mean that she will always hate being naked. Being wet, such as when a nappy has leaked, may cause crying. Obviously, on a cold day you must wrap your baby well – use as many layers as you would for yourself.

Illness

Likely type of cry Could be either intermittent or insistent; the crying may sound different to the usual cries; high-pitched and whining is a common description; maybe whimpering or a weaker cry than normal.
Other possible signs Obvious signs include wheezing, diarrheoa, pallor of skin, unusual drowsiness, loss of tone. A feverish baby may be hot to touch.
What to do This isn't meant to be a health manual, so consult your *Birth to Five* book, NHS Direct (0845 4647 – 24 hours), your doctor or health visitor if you suspect illness. We all worry that our babies might be ill when they cry a lot, but fever, pallor and floppiness are more reliable signs.

Pain or Discomfort

Likely type of cry Sudden, shrill, very loud in acute situation.
Other possible signs Some obvious discomfort, such as in a minor accident.
What to do Bumps are pretty inevitable as soon as babies start learning to manouevre themselves around. Usually the crying miraculously ceases after a quick cuddle and when you divert their attention.

Whether babies suffer from headaches and growing pains is not known for sure. Relatively little is spoken about the possibilities of after-pains from birth, such as when ventouse or forceps have been used, or from being in an awkward position in the uterus or birth canal. Consult a doctor if you suspect some kind of chronic pain or discomfort in your baby. Some osteopaths are qualified to treat certain types of physical problems in babies.

TEETHING

Likely type of cry All kinds, if you subscribe to the idea that teething causes pain and a host of other problems.

Other possible signs Dribbling, trying to chew everything, red cheeks (although dribbling and chewing can also be attributed to babies' oral exploration of the world, and red cheeks may be put down to skin irritation).

What to do Teething is regarded by many parents as a big source of misery for young children. But few of today's babycare experts subscribe to the idea that the emergence of teeth causes babies nearly as much discomfort and pain as popularly believed. They argue that unexplained crying is too often put down to "teething", while other problems, such as illness, tiredness or hunger, are overlooked. Certainly, the idea that teething causes side effects such as colds, diarrhoea and fever is discredited by health professionals and virtually all modern babycare manuals. If your child often goes through grumpy phases, this might be more of a personality trait than a direct link to teeth coming through. On the other hand, the manufacturers of teething rings, teething gels and homeopathic remedies would support the idea that the emergence of teeth can cause pain. One way or the other, teething pain is a bit like colic – whether your baby is really suffering from it or not may not be as important as being able to give the unexplained crying a name.

Consult a health professional if there's a very definite problem inside your baby's mouth – such as swollen, bleeding gums – that doesn't clear up quickly with the help of teething gels etc.

ANGER, FRUSTRATION AND IRRITABILITY

Likely type of cry Sudden onset or quickly building to insistent, loud screams. Might be worse some days for no apparent reason (like in adults).

Other possible signs Some obvious annoyance, such as not being allowed or not having the ability to do something, maybe quivering, going rigid or stamping in the older baby. Throwing themselves to the ground.

What to do In older babies and toddlers, anger, frustration and tantrums are easy to identify, and the way you handle the situation will depend on the context. It's hard to say how much newborns get angry. Some people say that newborns don't actually cry from irritability at all. Whatever you think about this, don't fall into the trap of believing that your newborn is angry with you personally.

INSECURITY, CLINGINESS AND FEAR

Likely type of cry Crying if you leave the room or put the baby down.

Other possible signs Shyness with strangers, needing a lot of reassurance.

What to do This kind of crying is also easily identifiable in older babies and toddlers and may happen in phases. How best to respond is quite an issue in babycare politics. The proponents of "attachment parenting" (see p91) say that babies naturally feel insecure and will do best if in near-constant physical contact with their parents, including in bed. By contrast, others say that babies can and should learn to be independent some of the time, for their own benefit and yours. In practice, most parents try out different ways of dealing with this according to the situation at the time. It's part of the individual relationship you develop together.

BOREDOM

Likely type of cry Intermittent.

Other possible signs Alert and responsive, maybe straining to move into a different position or manipulate nearby objects.

What to do Your baby's periods of alertness when she is well-fed and interested in her surroundings and not sleepy will quickly increase. A bored cry or cry for companionship will be easily stopped if you speak to her or do something different with her, or give her something new to look at or even just place her so she can see you engaged in some activity. She may want to be in a different position, so experiment with holding her upright, lying her on her belly (when she is wakeful), or in a baby chair.

If your attempts to interest her in different things work only for a few minutes before she starts to cry again then there is more likely to be some other reason for the crying, such as hunger or tiredness – you are merely diverting her attention.

"TALKING"

Likely type of cry Not really crying – maybe gentle, intermittent noises, cooing, an increasing range of vocalizing.

Other possible signs Alert, relaxed, lots of eye contact.

What to do Not every sound uttered by your baby is a cry, though in the very early days you may perhaps be too nervous or too tired to notice. Naturally, as the weeks go by, the "talking" becomes ever more exciting and rewarding. Help develop the range of sounds by singing, chatting and making noises, such as animal noises. Imitate the baby's sounds. You may feel silly doing it at first, but studies show that babies can respond well to "baby talk" from birth.

Comforts for the Newborn

An older child might stop crying the moment you enter the room or pick him up, but a newborn usually needs more tactile comforts for longer. When you can't fathom out why your well-fed young baby is crying, try these age-old ways of comforting that parents have employed through generations.

Sucking Comforts

Many babies carry on sucking the nipple for sheer pleasure long after they have filled up on milk (see p138). You might find you like this in the early days when you are happy to rest with your babe-in-arms. But a lot of mothers find comfort sucking on their breasts rather onerous as the weeks go by, and it can become a problem if your baby starts to rely on nursing as the main way in which to fall asleep (see pp176–177).

Many parents offer dummies (comforters), but they can be problematic, too. For a start, you need to learn how to distinguish when the baby has fed enough but still wants to suck for comfort (see p138). In the early months you will need to sterilise dummies, which is a chore. Also bear in mind that if your baby starts to rely on sucking the dummy in order to sleep, you might have to keep popping it back in when it falls out, which will be another chore until the baby learns how to do this himself at about four or five months. Then again, that chore doesn't bother some parents in the difficult early months, when the primary goal is to stop the crying. The baby might be happy to expend energy sucking the dummy, then let it fall out the mouth when bored of it.

Some babies refuse dummies by spitting them out. Even babies who do like them sometimes refuse them. And some babies get hooked on dummies, wanting them virtually the whole time. This can impede the development of speech. There is also a certain snobbery against the use of dummies, especially in older children, because of the way it looks and the very association of the word "dummy"; this is why the word "comforter" is sometimes preferred. The age at which your baby becomes capable of putting the dummy back in his mouth is also when he might learn finger-sucking and thumb-sucking as a self-comfort. This might be less problematic than the use of dummies in the early years – few parents discourage thumb-sucking until a child is much older.

RHYTHMIC MOVEMENTS AND SOUNDS

Rocking, dancing, pacing up and down with your babe-in-arms or resting on your shoulder, rubbing and patting the back gently, going for a walk, going for a drive, pushing the pram backwards and forwards, sitting in a rocking chair, using a rocking crib, playing white noise, singing lullabies, the sound of a heartbeat, any rhythmic music – they're all repetitive and lulling, and might work to soothe a crying baby. The theory is that they are reminiscent of the noises and movements of the uterine environment, though you may find that the rocking has to be faster than the speed at which you moved during pregnancy!

The main thing to watch out with these kinds of tricks is not to let something like rocking, which requires a lot of intervention on your part, become a part of actual sleep conditioning (see pp176–178). Use comforts such as these as a way of soothing a crying baby, but not too regularly as a deliberate way of inducing sleep, not after the early weeks anyway.

SKIN-TO-SKIN AND SOFT COMFORTS

You probably adore holding your baby next to your bare skin, though perhaps not for hours on end. While some people say that parents should carry their babies as much as possible (see p91), others say that babies can suffer stress from being over-handled. Your growing relationship together will guide you as to how much cuddling and body contact is appropriate. Alternatives to the comfort of skin include soft, furry materials, sheepskins, big teddy bears etc. Once older babies start reaching out, they will love touching their own bellies and genitals. Some get attached to a soft object – a particular blanket or cuddly toy perhaps, which are also referred to as "comforters".

SWADDLING AND SHUTTING OUT THE WORLD

Newborn babies have little control over their limbs and have a "startle" reflex that can disturb their own sleep. Swaddling – wrapping securely in a blanket so that the limbs can't flail around – is a time-honoured method. It helps to shut out external stimuli as well as being a tactile comfort. It doesn't require your constant intervention, either, so is not a problematic part of sleep conditioning. Other ways of shutting out the world include dimming or turning off the lights and reducing the noise level rather than using rhythmic noises and movements. If you have tried rocking etc but your baby is still upset, it could actually be because of the stimuli and stress of sensory bombardment. As an alternative, try swaddling and putting the baby to bed in a darkened, quiet room for a while to see if that helps. Just make sure you don't overheat the baby – each wrap of the swaddling blanket represents a layer (see p196).

WHO'S FOR SWADDLING?
Some people regard swaddling as primitive or even cruel. Of the popular babycare gurus, Penelope Leach and Gina Ford are for it; Miriam Stoppard is against it. The editor found that swaddling helped her own baby daughter to settle in the first three months or so. It looked odd to see her tiny form bundled up, but not in a cruel way.

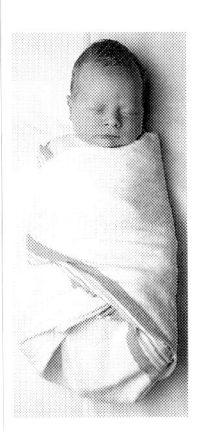

Typical Patterns of Baby Behaviour

There is a wide normal range of crying, waking, sleeping and feeding patterns in babies. By the time babies are a year old, the variations between individuals are not so marked as they are in the first six months. Here, **Robin Barker** summarizes the most common normal variations of healthy, well-fed babies in their first year.

ABOUT ROBIN BARKER
The author of this section is Australia's most popular baby-care expert. For more about her approach, see p81.

Why Talk About Typical Patterns?

Understanding the normal patterns of sleeping, feeding, crying etc in babies can be reassuring and helpful whether you are following a babycare regime as touted by the latest babycare expert or whether you are muddling along following your own instincts. Or perhaps, like most of us, you are doing a bit of both. Sometimes baby patterns can be changed to fit in with the adult lifestyle, sometimes they can't.

For the sake of clarity, this section is divided into age bands. You may not see such clear demarcations as this, but you should certainly notice a difference within the bands, such as at three weeks, seven weeks, eleven weeks, four months and so on.

Birth to Six Weeks

Sleeping Newborn babies get the amount of sleep they need (see p168) within a wide variation. Total sleep varies from 9 to 18 hours every 24 hours in six to eight sleeps. Most common is 12 to 14 hours every 24 hours. Many babies start out sleeping and eating in very regular patterns and may sleep regularly and for relatively long periods in the first two to three weeks.

Crying Sleeping and crying are inextricably linked. In the early months and to some extent during the whole of the first year, the less babies sleep, the more they cry. In the first two to three weeks many babies sleep a lot, the crying periods don't last long and are often easy to resolve. Most babies are only happy to be awake for relatively short periods of time before they start to cry. The younger they are the shorter the time they are happy to be up. Babies who sleep only nine hours every 24 are almost certainly going to cry more than babies who sleep 18 hours every 24. When they are healthy and well fed this does not harm them, but naturally life is difficult for the family, particularly the mother. Sometimes things can be done to help the baby sleep more and longer on his own and sometimes they can't. Most babies cry less when they are held in close body contact with another human.

Feeding The number of breastfeeds every 24 hours varies from six to eight. More is fine as long as mother is happy about breastfeeding frequently; less than six is usually not enough to maintain the milk supply. Some feeds are close together, others further apart. Trying to feed strictly every four hours works for some mothers and babies but generally a more flexible approach is needed. At least two night feeds is the norm.

With bottle-feeding, six to eight bottles every 24 hours are needed with appropriate amounts of infant formula (150ml per kilo of body weight). Bottle-fed babies, like breastfed babies, drink variable amounts and may have some feeds close together and others further apart.

Digestion The early poo (meconium), a greenish black sticky substance, gradually changes over the first few days until the colourful array of bowel motions start to appear. It is normal for breastfed babies to poo many times a day in the first six weeks in a variety of colours from lettuce green to pumpkin yellow. Some breasfed babies may only have one good poo every other day. Breastfed poo is always soft. Babies established on formula usually do a dark, sticky, more formed poo that looks like plasticine.

Burping and farting are normal functions of the human body from birth to death, and all babies fart very loudly and very well from the moment they arrive. The frequency, loudness and smelliness of their baby's farts often astound parents, especially in the first few weeks. Burping is something babies do naturally when they need to. The burping ritual that goes on in Western culture is by and large unnecessary although I acknowledge that it is very satisfying to hear a baby burp (I enjoy it too).

It is normal for healthy babies to vomit and regurgitate their food. The amount varies from a splat on your shoulder (a posset) after a feed to a great gush of milk onto the floor. About half of all babies vomit enough to worry their parents and complicate normal living. A small number of babies never do either. Vomiting and posseting generally doesn't start until two or three weeks after birth. While it is advisable to have any vomiting investigated if you are unsure of the cause, the majority of healthy vomiters have no ill effects from their vomiting.

Typical Patterns of Baby Behaviour (Robin Barker)

Possible Unsettled Phase

Between three and six weeks many babies start to behave quite erratically – sleeping less and crying more at times when it is difficult to work out what's the matter. This erratic behaviour can last until around three months, sometimes longer. In healthy, well-fed babies it is more likely to be due to adjustment to the strange world they find themselves in than to "colic", wind or "reflux" (heartburn).

Six to Eight Weeks

Sleeping The most common 24-hour sleeping and waking pattern now is: one five- to six-hour sleep (if you're lucky during the night – often the bulk of the sleep is before 1am); one or two three-hourly sleeps; several two-hourly sleeps; up to five or six hours of catnapping, interspersed with wakefulness and crying (the unsettled period).

About eight out of ten babies have one unsettled period every 24 hours varying from two to five hours. The unsettled period is a session of unexplained crying, usually in the evening, sometimes between 1am and 4am. The unsettled period continues until three months for many babies.

However, some babies do none of the above and eat and sleep in a predictable routine.

Feeding Six to eight feeds every 24 hours continue. Most babies need to feed at least six times every 24 hours to maintain the milk supply while being exclusively breastfed. A four-hourly schedule is possible for some babies but most breastfed babies need more flexibility. Some babies will be happy with longer intervals between breastfeeds by the time they are eight weeks old, but individual babies differ widely in this regard. One to three feeds, sometimes more, during the night is normal (see "sleeping through" in the eight to twelve weeks age band and What is a Settled Sleep Pattern? on p169).

Formula-fed babies will need five to eight bottles every 24 hours, with appropriate amounts of infant formula (150mls per kilo of body weight). Babies having formula may fall into a routine with longer intervals between feeds than breastfed babies, but this is variable from baby to baby. One to two feeds through the night is normal.

Digestion Breastfed babies' poo varies from one to six or more a day in a variety of colours. Some breastfed babies have several days between good poos. This is normal and needs no treatment. Breastfed babies rarely get constipated (hard poo). Their poo is always soft even if they don't go for a few days. Many breastfed babies grunt, groan, go red in the face or even cry at times when they do a poo. This is usually due to the unusual sensation, not wind, "colic" or reflux.

Bottle-fed babies usually do a firmer poo than breastfed babies, darker colour, one or more a day. If babies having formula go two or more days without a poo simple treatment is needed, for example, extra water. Many formula-fed babies also grunt, groan, go red in the face or even cry at times when they do a poo, due to the unusual sensation. Occasionally it is due to hard poo (like a rock) which needs treatment.

All babies burp and fart as they need to. At times they show what appears to be distress to these normal body functions – again this is more likely to be because of the weird sensation than because of "gut problems". Most babies continue to bring up splats of milk with their burps. If it comes up soon after it goes down it looks like milk. If it comes up sometime later it is partly digested and looks curdled. Vomiting is common.

A small number of babies neither vomit nor posset.

Related developmental milestone at four to eight weeks The baby stares at mother's face, smiles and coos; grasps a finger placed in hand; stops crying when picked up and spoken to; and turns to the sound of a soothing voice.

Eight to Twelve Weeks

Sleeping and crying By three months many babies are in a much more predictable sleeping and waking patterns. The unsettled period has passed and there is much less crying. However, some babies continue to be unpredictable, sleep little and cry a lot. This is usually within the normal range. Occasionally specific medical/feeding problems are diagnosed, but often no reason is ever found for their unpredictable behaviour.

The most common 24-hour sleeping and waking pattern now is: one five- to six-hour sleep (at night, usually in the first half of the night); one three- to four-hour sleep (early hours of the morning); three one-and-a-half- to two-hour sleeps in the day (a common regime suggested by baby experts is "up one-and-a-half to two hours, down one-and-a-half to two hours", which works well for some babies but is an impossible goal for others).

But...common variations include: no long sleep – baby continues to wake every two to three hours through the night; catnaps only during the day – 20 to 40 minutes – impossible to get baby to sleep for longer periods despite fevered attempts to "resettle" when baby wakes.

Some babies will go to sleep on their own, some will go to sleep after crying for short periods, some need to be fed, rocked, patted, nursed to sleep.

Typical Patterns of Baby Behaviour (Robin Barker)

"Sleeping through" refers to the stage when babies start to put themselves back to sleep in the night without waking their parents. The age at which they do this varies tremendously and is a cause of great angst among parents.

Common variations include: baby takes a late evening feed (between 8pm and 11pm) and an early morning feed (1am to 4am). Roughly six out of ten babies stop waking for one of these feeds between six and twelve weeks. It is often the earlier feed. Babies generally have their longest, deepest sleep before 1am. About two or three babies in ten continue to wake and cry every two to three hours through the night for the whole of the first six months.

Some babies sleep 10 hours a night from six to eight weeks of age. This is more likely to come from within the baby than to have anything to do with the mother's care or the advice of a guru. The relationship between food and night waking is extremely variable. Sometimes extra food in the day or evening improves night waking, but more often than not it makes no difference.

Feeding Six to eight (or more) breastfeeds continues. Unlike formula feeding, where the amount in the bottle increases and the number of bottles gets less as the baby grows, at least six breastfeeds need to be given every 24 hours in order to maintain sufficient milk supply. The number of breastfeeds every 24 hours does not change until the baby is established on solids or starts having formula as well as breastmilk.

Five to seven bottles every 24 hours for formula-fed babies (150mls per kilo of body weight).

Digestion Around three months, about half of all breastfed babies store up their poo and only go once in a while – the time varies from a couple of days up to three weeks. This is normal. The longer the poo is stored the smellier their farts become. This is also normal and needs no treatment. When the poo comes it is mammoth: bad luck if you're out and about.

With bottle-fed babies it's nice to see a good poo every day or so as babies having formula can get constipated, which is distressing for them. If necessary extra water or juice can be given to keep their poo soft.

By three months most babies are showing less distress with burping, farting, possetting and vomiting as they get used to their body functions. Possetting continues, and about a half of all babies vomit, some copiously. Most are "happy vomiters" with no ill effects from their throwing up.

Related developmental milestones Visually very alert; follows the parent's face; plays with hands – fist constantly in the mouth (this is not "hunger" or "teething", but normal sensory-motor development); lots of talking noises; loves to be played with and talked to.

Three to Six Months

Sleeping and crying Sleep patterns are similar to previous section. Between three and six months the majority of babies slowly become more predictable and a pattern or routine emerges. Feeding and sleeping times still might vary from day to day for many babies. Others will be in a strict routine.

A word about routines Routines suit adults as it means we can plan our day. Routines also have the potential to allow parents to schedule some time off for themselves and, if the routine is working, get more sleep at night. Babies do not need routines until they are mobile and becoming toddlers at which time routines are needed for their stability, security and safety and parental sanity. Some babies slip into a routine almost from birth, others need more time and flexibility and will not be in a predictable routine until somewhere between six and nine months.

"Strict" routines can be difficult to maintain in the first year, especially the first six months. Illness, holidays, moving house or visitors can all play havoc with strict routines. Keeping one means structuring your life exactly around your baby's schedule, which limits your movements and can mean putting up with an intolerable amount of crying for no constructive purpose other than to live by the clock. Babies who are in strict routines from birth do not grow up to be better people.

The majority of crying, unsettled babies who don't sleep much become happier and better sleepers somewhere between four and six months. A few babies remain poor sleepers and grumblebums for the whole of the first year. Babies, like all of us, don't stay the same day in and day out. Sudden erratic changes are common and 'bad' days happen, often for no apparent reason.

Night waking variations: about six out of ten babies are sleeping eight to twelve hours at night by six months of age. The remaining four are still waking once, twice or more every night or some nights. Many babies "sleep through" at eight weeks only to start waking once or twice a night again between four and six months. This rarely has anything to do with food and is more related to developmental factors such as a greater awareness of the world around them, new body movements such as rolling over, sitting up, kicking bedclothes off.

Feeding Six or more breastfeeds every 24 hours or four to five bottles a day (120ml per kilo of body weight). Most babies do not need food other than

Typical Patterns of Baby Behaviour (Robin Barker)

breastmilk or formula until sometime between four and six months. All babies respond to solids in their own way. Here are a few common variations: loves the food, eats anything offered; takes the food well initially then loses interest; initially completely refuses all food; loves some things, refuses others; keeps refusing food throughout most of the first year; will not eat slush, eventually eats only finger food.

Digestion It is common for breastfed babies to become constipated (hard poo) once they are having regular solids. The main offenders are rice cereal and banana, and if this happens their diets need adjusting to accommodate the constipation. Happy vomiters usually keep vomiting away. Introduction of solids does very little to stop the vomiting other than to make it multi-coloured rather than white. The vomiting may reduce to some extent when the baby is able to sit alone (six to nine months).

Related developmental milestones at six months Good head control; some babies are sitting; rolling (probably); passes things from one hand to another; watches falling objects; puts everything in mouth; reaches out and grabs things.

Six to Twelve Months

Sleeping and crying This is the age where a more predictable routine starts to kick in for the babies who have been all over the shop with their sleeping, crying and eating. The most common 24-hour sleeping and waking pattern now is: 10 to 12 hours sleep through the night; two to three daytime sleeps (number of day sleeps depends on the time the baby wakes in the morning), varying from one to two hours. Between nine and twelve months most babies have two daytime sleeps.

But...common variations include: two or more night wakings, especially between 1am and 5am. At least half of all babies wake anytime from 4:30am ready to start the day. Some babies continue to catnap in the day (20 to 40 minutes). This can be very difficult to do anything about and some parents find putting the suggested regimes into place to get the baby to sleep for longer periods are not worth the drama.

Night waking, early morning waking and daytime catnapping do not hurt babies but obviously can be exhausting for parents. In my experience it is usually difficult to do anything about catnapping or early morning waking but night waking patterns can be changed for many babies by doing what is commonly known as "control crying" (see pp179–180). If the parents are reluctant to do this or try it and find it doesn't work for them then they have to

---

ROBIN BARKER'S SUGGESTED WEANING STRATEGY
• Early morning – breast or bottle feed
• Mid morning (any time from 9am to 11am) – rice cereal with cooked fruit plus breast/bottle ("breakfast")
• Early afternoon (any time from 1pm to 3pm) – blended vegetables (add meat and chicken from six months) plus breast/bottle ("lunch")
• Early evening (any time from 4.30pm to 7pm) – yoghurt and fruit or mashed banana or avocado/cottage cheese blended or chicken broth with rice cereal plus breast/bottle ("dinner").
• Late evening – breast or bottle (if needed)

learn to live with the night waking, which may continue until the baby is three years old. Many parents in this situation find that sharing the family bed works best.

Feeding Number of breastfeeds varies from three to eight depending on amount of solids being eaten, night waking and the mother's breastfeeding philosophy. Some babies have water or juice from a bottle, others drink from a cup (highly recommended). Many breastfed babies are weaned by 12 months – many straight onto cow's milk in a cup.

Number of formula bottles varies from three to four (200–180mls three times a day after meals is sufficient). By 12 months, two a day is recommended with an aim of stopping the bottles as soon as possible into the second year. Formula labelled "suitable from birth" is fine for the whole of the first year. "Follow-on" formula labelled "suitable for babies over six months" is a marketing term – the extra bulk of "follow-on" milk is not essential when you start weaning. Toddler formula is another marketing ploy and not recommended by the majority of health authorities. Cow's milk in a cup is the best option.

By nine months of age babies can be offered a wide variety of food including finger food once they are sitting well on their own. Eating patterns are similar to those in previous section. Some fussy eaters will now be eating, others remain reluctant until around a year, still others are fussy for the rest of their lives! As babies approach toddlerhood many formerly good eaters suddenly start refusing their vegetables. Toddlers are renowned for their fussy eating habits.

Digestion It is normal to see recycled food in the poo once babies start eating chunkier food. Most of the happy vomiters are still doing it! There is often an increase in the vomiting when the baby learns to crawl. As he is horizontal to the ground for much of the time the regurgitated food tends to slide out. All but one in 20 of the happy vomiters will have stopped vomiting by 12 months.

Related developmental milestones at nine months Sits alone; attempting to crawl or actually crawling or maybe even walking; pulls to standing; picks up small things with finger and thumb; holds food and chews it; bangs two blocks together.

At 12 months Crawls, cruises while holding onto furniture, walks (some still just sit); refined pincer grasp with finger and thumb; points with index finger; holds a spoon; tips things out of containers; understands the meaning of many concepts and words as well as simple instructions.

A BIG CHAPTER ABOUT FEEDING

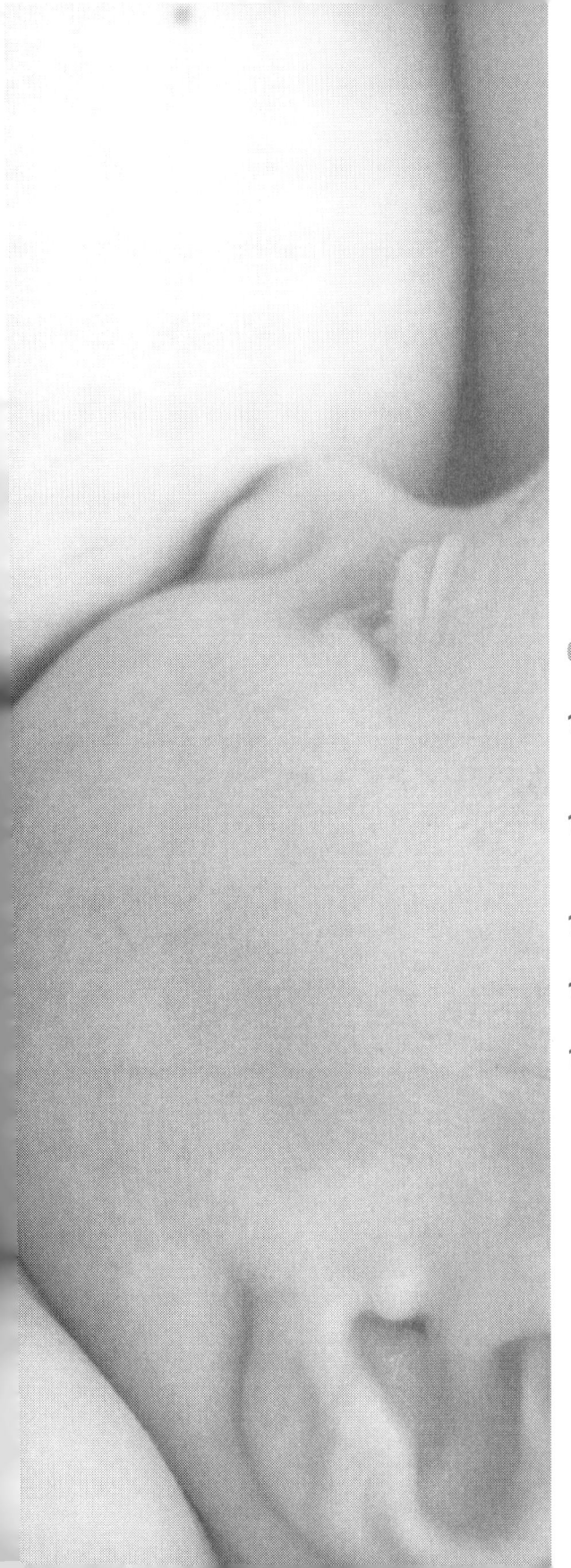

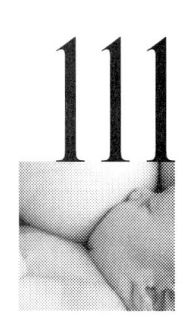

Contents

112 A Feeding Summary for the First Year

114 How Breastfeeding Works

122 What's in Milk?

124 Breastfeeding Politics

134 Feeding Rhythms

A Feeding Summary for the First Year

Feeding your child will preoccupy much of your time from birth (and for evermore), and almost certainly will be a source of both pleasure and frustration. You will also have to pick your way through the different attitudes to milk and weaning. Nutritional information has varied over the decades - the Birth to Five manual is a good place to start for up-to-date advice.

WHAT IS WEANING?
The word "weaning" is used to mean all of these things: moving from breast to bottles; from breastmilk to formula; the introduction of solids alongside milk; and from formula to standard cow's milk.

The First Four to Six Months

Milk is all your baby needs up to the age of four to six months. After this, milk remains the number one food, but you can start to introduce others alongside it. Don't leave the introduction of other foods longer than six months, because your baby then starts to require more nutrition than milk alone can provide. This advice of solely milk for four to six months is standard now, but it wasn't always so – the start of weaning was often three months or earlier, until it was discovered that babies' digestive enzymes aren't mature until about 16 weeks (that's for a full-term baby – a premature baby will need more time just on milk).

Ideally, the milk your baby consumes should be yours because it has far more health benefits than any other milk. You probably know this already, but the benefits are summarized on pp122–123. In late pregnancy and the first few days following birth, human breasts produce a creamy yellow substance called colostrum, which has a great concentration of immunity-boosting cells. There's not much volume to colostrum, but your baby's frequent suckling on it will help to "bring your milk in" a few days later. This strange phenomenon will leave your breasts full, heavy and possibly lumpy and dripping with the proper milk.

Getting breastfeeding established into a good, pain-free rhythm is a bit of an art, which is why there are reams of advice on the subject and also why it can be an early source of joy and despair for mothers. But if breastfeeding works well, the baby needs no other supplement of any kind, not even water, for four to six months, because the breasts continually adjust the constituents of the milk in response to the baby's requirements. When breastfeeding doesn't work out well, mothers usually start supplementing breastmilk with formula baby milk. Formula is usually based on cow's milk with added vitamins and other substances. Much of the rest of this chapter covers breastfeeding and feeding rhythms in more detail.

Expect to feed a minimum of six to eight times in 24 hours (possibly more) for the first couple of months, whether breast or bottle. As time goes by you can encourage the baby to take in more during the daytime feeds, easing the burden on you for night feeds (see p144 and the Sleep chapter).

SIX MONTHS TO ONE YEAR

A few teaspoons of mashed or puréed foods each day are all that are needed for at least a month after you start to wean onto "solids" alongside the mainstay of milk. Such foods are as much for your baby's experience as extra nutrition. The standard advice is to start off with simple fruits and vegetables. As the weeks go by you can try a wider variety of foods (see also p108).

As with what adults eat, fresh food is superior to processed baby foods both for nutrition and taste. Babies can be encouraged to deal with lumpy foods from an early age – there's no need to wait until they have teeth, which was the tendency in previous decades. Moreover, the ages of about nine to twelve months are considered critical in introducing a variety of taste and texture – otherwise your baby may become hooked on bland, puréed foods. Babies have a gag reflex, which helps them learn what consistency they have to chomp the food to. The only stuff to avoid giving until the back teeth have grown is small hard foods that need a lot of grinding, like nuts.

Babies increasingly show preferences and disdain for different foods from the moment you start to introduce them and throughout childhood. Again, this is a potential source of pleasure and irritation for you. Nothing is simple, and what most parents do is continually broaden the variety of foods so that a reasonably balanced diet and interesting range of tastes and textures are on offer, whilst also keeping to some favourites for simplicity.

Feeding is time-consuming and messy – preparing separate meals three times a day, spooning it into your baby's mouth and clearing up the ensuing chaos. In addition, your baby will still be drinking milk and probably snacking in between formal meals. All in all, the more skills your baby develops to hold the food and grapple with chunks, the happier you both will be. Within a few months you will be able to share some of the same meals, thus easing the workload.

Breastmilk or formula milk feeding can stabilise at about a pint a day, including milk products such as cheese and yoghurt. It is only after a year that you can introduce normal full-fat milk (not semi-skimmed). By the age of one year, according to the *Birth to Five* manual, your child is allowed any foods except shellfish (food poisoning risk) and peanuts (allergy and inhalation risk).

TOP BOOKS ON FEEDING

• *The Birth to Five manual from your midwife has a good section on weaning.*

• *Annabel Karmel's recipes and advice about weaning are very popular, such as in her New Complete Baby and Toddler Meal Planner (Ebury Press 2001) and Feeding Your Baby and Toddler (Dorling Kindersley 1999).*

• *Nigella Lawson has a great chapter on feeding babies and small children in her How to Eat book.*

• *See also the breastfeeding books listed on p130.*

How Breastfeeding Works

It helps to know something about how breastfeeding works so you can feel confident from the start. On pp122–123 is more detail about what's in human and formula milk. The important subject of breastfeeding politics is covered on pp124–133, and the intricacies of finding a good feeding rhythm are on pp134–151.

How the "Mammary Glands" Gear Up

From the moment your body registers that it is pregnant, hormonal signals head for your breasts and start preparing the milk ducts for action. They continue to develop for nine months, and towards the end of pregnancy you might notice a slight discharge of a creamy substance. This isn't mature milk, but a much thicker and concentrated milk called colostrum. If you cup your fingers around the breast, above the areola, and squeeze and draw down towards the nipple in a milking action (not on the nipple itself, which will probably hurt), you might be able to express a few drops of colostrum before birth. Hand expressing is a useful skill. But don't worry if you can't see any colostrum yet.

The sudden loss of the placenta after birth triggers hormone changes, with a massive surge to your mammary glands. There will be a few days whilst your body adjusts to these changes, during which the baby's frequent suckling of colostrum will stimulate your milk ducts and give your baby's immune system a huge boost.

Some babies seem to know instinctively how to "latch on" and suck away at a breast, but many may need some help. You can help by positioning the baby at a precise angle on the breast (see tips about positioning, opposite).

When the mature milk – a much runnier and voluminous liquid – "comes in" two to seven days later you may experience a sudden sensation of fullness. Your breasts may be literally a bra size bigger (or more) in the space of a few hours and feel tightly packed, maybe a bit lumpy and probably uncomfortable until the baby empties them. It will be important to find a good rhythm of breastfeeding (see pp134–151) partly to avoid your breasts frequently becoming engorged, which can lead to great discomfort. Your baby may need more help to latch on to your fuller breasts once the milk has come in.

A Big Chapter About Feeding

"Rooting" and "Latching On"

There are a lot of misunderstandings about the mechanics of breastfeeding. After all, you can't see exactly what is happening. It's useful to learn how a baby sucks and what is going on behind your nipple when you come to help the baby "latch on". Your baby will not get much milk by sucking at your nipple as if it were a straw, and your nipples will soon suffer if you let your baby attempt this.

When we suck on a straw we just use our lips and long in-breaths to provide suction. By contrast, when babies get going properly on a breast, they use their tongues in a powerful back and forth rippling rhythm, which shoots four or five fine jets (as opposed to one jet) of milk into the roof of the mouth. One of the main things you might have to do is help the baby get more of the nipple into its mouth. Women with relatively small nipples should be able to get the whole areola in; women with larger areolas should aim to get as much in as possible. If the baby just latches on to the narrow part of the nipple, the pinching will cause you pain. If you are not convinced of this, try tweaking the end of your nipple between finger and thumb – probably very sensitive. Now try further up, by the wide areola – less sensitive. Now beyond the areola – nothing like the same sensation.

To take in this much nipple, your baby needs to open its mouth very wide. Typically, you might find that the baby starts "rooting" – opening and twisting the mouth in search of something – but doesn't open wide enough or long enough for you to get much areola in before clamping onto the end of the nipple. In fact, this scenario is proof that both newborn babies and new mothers are a crazy mix of half-formed instincts. You are probably instinctively trying to push the breast into the mouth; the baby is instinctively trying to suck on something. Yet it may not gel together. What you may need are some tips about positioning from other breastfeeding mothers.

Tips About Positioning

A full feed can take a long time (see p137), and you're going to be doing it many times a day, so get into a well-supported, comfortable position beforehand. Your arms as well as your back need support. A popular way is sitting upright with a big cushion on the lap to help support the babe-in-arms; or lying on one side with lots of cushions to support your own head, neck and back. Experiment to see what feels comfortable. Women who have just had a caesarian may not be able to sit up normally, but with extra props should be able to breastfeed, perhaps lying down.

The next element is the baby's positioning against you. Perhaps the most "instinctive" position is to let the baby lie face up in your arms with the head

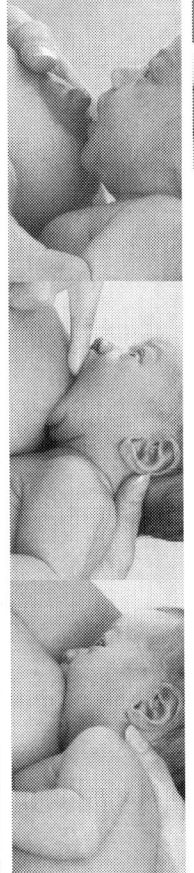

Good positioning will minimise pain for you and ensure your baby gets the milk easily. Note how low the baby's jaw drops in order to latch on.

How Breastfeeding Works

roughly positioned below your nipple, but in fact this is problematic with a newborn baby. The reason for this is that the newborn will have to twist her neck to latch onto the breast, but this isn't easy because she has little or no control over her head muscles at this stage. If she does manage to latch on, she will have a kink in her throat, and so be unable to suck straight or swallow properly. Also, your breast may be pulled at an odd angle, perhaps inhibiting the flow of milk. So avoid this position even if it looks kind of ok.

The baby's whole body has to be parallel with yours if you are to avoid the neck twist. The easiest thing to do is just make sure the baby's tummy is pressed against yours. "Tummy to mummy" is the mantra of some breastfeeding classes.

Gather the baby belly to belly with you, and with her nose – not mouth – parallel with your nipple. The reason for this one is so that once she opens her mouth and latches on, her head will be very slightly tipped back, automatically widening the throat. Think of the way in which you might tip your head back a little to glug from a bottle of pop.

So far, so good. But perhaps your baby's mouth isn't open, or not open very wide. To encourage the rooting reflex, gently brush the baby's cheek against your nipple a few times, "teasingingly". Hopefully she will then suddenly open wide for a couple of seconds. Bring her right in and on firmly, making sure that the areola goes deep into the mouth. As soon as she feels the breast and nipple against her tongue she will probably start sucking.

Notice that the advice with each stage is that you bring the baby to you, not that you bend and push your body at the baby. If you do the latter, you're very likely to end up hunched over for long minutes, which will be bad for your shoulders and back. So the full, rather fey, breastfeeding mantra is "tummy to mummy; baby to breast; and nose to nipple".

TIP: Positioning will become less critical as the weeks go by – your baby will soon get used to feeding and start to gain control of neck muscles, while at the same time your breasts will probably adapt to the sucking and so become less sensitive.

TIP: If you have another child, don't forget that positioning will be critical again.

THE MILK "LET-DOWN"

So now you've got a good position and the baby is latched on, but where is the milk? Indeed, our breasts aren't like milk bottles, or gravity would make them constantly stream the stuff to the ground. The milk is in the ducts awaiting a release signal. Your baby's sucking is the main prompt, and a signal will go to and from your brain to tell your milk ducts to "let-down". You probably won't feel in control of this reflex. What you might feel after a few seconds of your baby sucking is a sudden sensation in your breasts of fluid rushing through narrow channels. It may feel like a tingling or slight burning sensation – for many women it is a bit unpleasant, maybe a touch painful at first, or, for some unfortunate women, very painful. But after a few more seconds any tingling or

A Big Chapter About Feeding

unpleasantness should dissipate. If the feed continues to be painful, there is perhaps something wrong – maybe the baby is sucking on the end of the nipple instead of above the areola. Once the baby is well latched on and the milk is flowing, breastfeeding really should not be painful. If it is, consult a midwife, health visitor or specialist breastfeeding counsellor (see p130).

You may be aware of this "let-down" reflex with colostrum, but if not, you might become more aware once your milk comes in. And as if the milk "let-down" isn't weird enough when you experience it for the first time, the brain simultaneously sends a message to your womb to contract. In the first 30 seconds or so of your baby feeding, you may feel flutters or slight cramps (or big cramps if you are unfortunate) in your lower abdomen. If you find this sensation unpleasant, at least take comfort to know that it is doing good – the quicker your womb contracts to its pre-pregnancy size, the quicker your reproductive system will recover. Also, the cramps are not necessarily always going to be painful. The uterine contractions related to the milk let-down take place in a similar zone to the spasms of orgasm – of course not the same, but consider them related. Such cramps will probably subside after some seconds as the baby continues feeding and emptying your breast. After a few weeks of breastfeeding, when your womb is nearly back to its old size, the crampiness might be more like fluttering. And it appears to be the case that some women do not feel such uterine spasms at all.

The let-down reflex has to happen during expressing, too, and this is when you might become more aware of the subconscious brain's involvement. If you are stressed, the let-down reflex can be inhibited. Women who express a lot might have odd occasions when the milk just will not flow (see p145–147) – perhaps it's being done in too much of a hurry, or the baby-less setting with an artificial pump is the inhibiting factor. For the let-down reflex not to happen when it is your actual baby on the breast is less likely, but not unknown. Consult someone appropriate if you think your baby is not getting much milk.

On a last note about the milk let-down, it will probably happen on both breasts, so either put a breast pad over the opposite one or have a cloth handy. There will be a free flow on the side that your baby is on, while the other one slowly drips. If the feeding stops for more than a few seconds, then resumes, you might feel a milder let-down reflex again.

TIP: If you leak in between feeds, this is perhaps the response of your breasts to half-conscious thoughts about feeding your baby or maybe to friction with clothing. It is most likely to happen when your breasts are quite full. If you press each nipple flat with the heel of your hand for a few moments, the drips should stop. Breast pads will help protect your bra.

Foremilk and Hindmilk

As with full-fat cow's milk, which you can see in a glass pint bottle has a creamy bit on top, human milk also comes in two consistencies. The runnier foremilk comes out of your breasts first, followed by the thick, creamy hindmilk (if you express an ounce or more and leave it to stand, you will see it separate into the two consistencies). The foremilk is the thirst-quencher; the hindmilk has the concentration of calories. Some foremilk will always be present in your breasts even when the baby has had a full feed – you are never entirely empty because the mammary glands keep replenishing it.

FINISHING A FEED

You will be able to see the baby's jaw and ear moving as he sucks. With a full feed, the sucking will probably be full force for many minutes, then begin to slow and eventually become intermittent. The standard advice is to let newborn babies feed for as long as they want, either until they loosen suction and turn away from the breast or fall asleep on it (see p137). Once the sucking has become intermittent, however, it can sometimes be difficult to tell just by looking whether the baby has finished or not, or if the sucking is continuing more for comfort and joy than for food. On the occasions when you want to finish the feed before the baby has stopped sucking, slide one finger into the corner of your baby's mouth to break the vacuum. Don't just try to pull baby and breast apart – your nipple might bear the brunt...

TIP: Lactation takes quite a lot of energy and fluid from your body, which may make you feel more thirsty than usual, especially in summer. Quench your thirst with water and have as many snacks as you like. Dehydration will only make you feel more tired.

THE CHANGING SUPPLY

Another important thing to know about breastfeeding is that your breasts continually adjust the quantity and quality of milk to roughly match your child's changing requirements. Supply is dependent on how often your baby feeds and how much he ingests, and each feed is a bit different in composition and quality.

The general advice from lactation specialists is to let your baby lead the way with feeds – whenever and for as long as he wants – and you can rely on your body to respond to the demand. (The term "demand feeding" is often used – see pp134–137.) Your milk will adjust to match the needs of anything from a premature baby to a one-year-old and beyond if need be. The demand-and-supply relationship is in some ways a wonderful, near-magical feature of breastfeeding, but it is also a factor that can complicate the early months of motherhood. The relationship with the child is symbiotic and intense.

For instance, if you miss one or more feeds in a row (say, by going out for a few hours while someone else feeds the baby), then you may become engorged followed by a drop in supply, unless you can express the excess while you are away from the baby. Many women successfully express on a regular basis, but not everyone finds it easy. The unpredictability of a newborn baby's feeding can be both alarming and mentally tiring for a new mother, who may find herself craving order. Very frequent feeds, every couple of hours around the clock, are quite normal in the early days. If you are exclusively breastfeeding (no formula), which is the ideal in the newborn period, then only you can do the feeds, including the night feeds (again, because of potential engorgement and drop in supply), which means that getting an unbroken stretch of more than a couple of hours of deep sleep may be impossible for some time to come. Some women have the ability to adapt to broken sleep without too much ill effect, breastfeeding half asleep in bed with the baby at night, and taking extra naps during the day to help make up the sleep. Others do not adapt well – their bodies and minds continue to suffer from ongoing sleep deprivation – and may find exclusive breastfeeding a living nightmare. If you find that the latter applies to you, then you have a difficult situation. Having someone stand in with a bottle of expressed milk or formula for some of the night feeds may enable you to sleep a longer stretch (so long as the baby is out of earshot). But you will become over-full with milk, and your body will lower the milk production to compensate. By a somewhat cruel twist of physiology, night feeds are the most efficient ones at boosting and maintaining milk supply because hormone levels are higher at night.

Breastfeeding and the demand-and-supply relationship usually takes a few weeks to establish (see p141). Once it does, though, you and your baby will have found a rhythm that keeps you both happy, your breasts won't be painful and any minor fluctuations in supply won't matter. However, when breastfeeding doesn't become established, noticeable fluctuations in supply can lead to worry and upset. Having too much milk can be uncomfortable (see engorgement below), and having too little for a prolonged time is one of the main reasons why mothers start supplementing with formula within a few days or weeks of birth. Low supply is looked at in more detail on p139.

TIP: Some of us have relatively sensitive nipples, so that even when positioning is correct there may be a certain level of soreness. On the whole, any such sensitivity is likely to decrease after a few weeks. Some women find that the calendula-based nipple creams (available from pharmacies) can help, in much the same way that hand creams might help if you have dry, chapped hands. However, some breastfeeding counsellors say that nipple creams have little more than a placebo effect. They won't help if your nipples are sore from poor positioning.

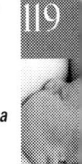

ENGORGEMENT

You'll probably experience the sensation of being over-full, or engorged, a few times, especially when your milk first comes in and you are still getting used to breastfeeding. It's not a pleasant sensation, but not necessarily painful – yet. Empty them as soon as possible, preferably with a normal feed. If that's not possible for some reason, hand express the excess on both sides until they feel more comfortable. Holding a warm cloth to them may help with expressing. Some people use chilled, crushed cabbage leaves (not on the nipple). If you leave breasts in an engorged state for long you risk blocked ducts, which are painful. Mastitis might then develop very quickly, giving you a fever. Feed and express to relieve all these problems, and consult a health visitor, doctor, etc if you have fever or pain that doesn't go when your breasts are emptied.

Some Stories About Breastfeeding

This small selection of stories shows how variable the experience of breastfeeding can be. There are also more views about the politics of breastfeeding on p133 and stories about feeding rhythms on pp149–151.

Rosalyn: "I really enjoyed breastfeeding from the start. The bonding between the two of us was out of this world, and the milk production itself fascinating. It's so much nicer than cow's milk – lovelier even than coconut milk. Luckily I didn't have many problems, maybe a few occasions when I suffered engorgement. Expressing was quite easy, too. She had nothing but breastmilk for four months, then we introduced formula. I continued breastfeeding morning and evening for another four months, during which my periods re-started. Then she got into a habit of snacking for a few seconds at a time, which became irritating. I was considering whether to continue, then one day she bit me. Some of my friends hadn't minded too much when their babies bit them, but to me this was the signal to stop."

Ruth: "It was very hard for the first two or three weeks. Just incredible, toe-curling, eye-watering soreness when the baby latched on. I still don't understand why it has to be so hard, after you've moved heaven and earth to get the baby out. After that, breastfeeding was fine, not painful, though perhaps a bit unwieldy. Feeding in public was never much fun, what with struggling with straps, and the baby not latching on. Also, I had huge, dangling boobs, compared with small-breasted women with tiny "pop on" babies. Mine was big and struggled. She stopped by herself at six months, just lost interest. I did miss it at first, but I feel more of an equal partner with her father now."

Justine: "The first few feeds weren't painful, but then my nipples became tender. Breastfeeding leaflets said that pain would stop 30 seconds into a feed, and this turned out to be true. The first time I fed in public was in a café with another breastfeeding mum for solidarity. It was never a problem to feed in public after that. I went back to work at six months and had intended to keep feeding morning and night, but sadly my milk dried up. For a few weeks I didn't feel like a mother anymore. I still really miss the closeness of feeding her."

Jo: "I used to have a poster of a Renaissance painting of Mary feeding the baby Jesus, which I ripped off the wall a week after the birth. My breasts were like footballs by then, and I was really worked up over breastfeeding. I couldn't bear to look down at him feeding from me – the whole act felt so crude and sordid. I kept thinking of vampires, of him sucking me dry. My sister came round to help, and that was when he started on bottles as I slept. Once he was fully onto bottles a week later I started to feel a lot better about things. Looking back, I know that I went mad for a while because of the breastfeeding. I can see why wet nurses were so popular in the past." (See also Jo's bonding story on p204.)

Alice: "Like many people my age (born in the late 1960s), I was bottle fed. And I have always been very fit and healthy. However, I personally found that breastfeeding has some big advantages over bottle-feeding. He dodged chicken-pox and colds while I was breastfeeding him; it helped me to lose weight; and it was good to have a food supply always on tap! The main disadvantage I found was that I was physically, and also therefore mentally, totally tied to the baby. I always felt a mild sense of panic whenever I was not with him, believing that he couldn't do without me. I'm sure this was linked to my breastfeeding him. Having stopped now, this feeling has disappeared. I view it as a positive benefit that he can get everything he needs without me. Other disadvantages were that I didn't always want to breastfeed – in front of male friends or relatives, for example. Also, I didn't like carrying around enormous boobs.

Whilst I think that breastfeeding is overall the best choice, I think that it is very wrong to make women feel guilty if they choose not to, as they are already coping with more than they've probably ever had to in their lives. I had a taste of this when I tried, and ultimately then gave up, expressing milk and felt like a failure for doing so. This really is a personal, not a political, issue."

Emma: "I had liked the idea of breastfeeding and wanted to try for as long as I could. It was a marvellous feeling to be able to feed my own baby, and he obviously enjoyed it so much. I had difficulties, though, and certainly didn't feel like I had enough milk to give him in the evenings. At two weeks, I started giving one bottle of formula at 11pm, to help him sleep longer in the night. After another few weeks I started topping him up with formula during daytime, too, and eventually gave up breastfeeding at about 10 weeks. It was a relief to stop, but I also felt guilty, as though I was taking away something he loved."

Annette: "In the beginning I found it to be very painful and had sore nipples. But I was determined to persevere, and after three days, when Annie and I had got more used to each other, the pain eased up. After a fortnight there was no discomfort at all, and I also took more care with making myself comfortable with cushions etc and ensuring she was in the correct position. I had wanted to breastfeed for at least three months, and managed four."

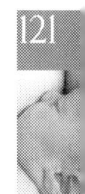

What's In Milk?

Milk is a fascinating substance, an essential part of mammalian reproduction. You'll start to produce the stuff in late pregnancy. Humans can survive on nothing other than their mothers' milk in the first six months or so of life outside the womb – not even extra water is needed.

Mammalian Milk

The mammary glands allow mammals to nurture their offspring to a high level of maturity before independence. In evolutionary terms, this is thought to be a key part of mammalian success. (Compare the sheltered life of a baby mammal able to receive full nourishment from its mother's milk with the dangerous life of a baby reptile that has to work out what to eat as soon as it hatches.)

Like other newborn mammals, humans cannot digest anything other than milk. This will soon change. From about four months of age, humans develop intestinal enzymes that allow them to digest simple plant matter. By seven or eight months, they can digest a wider range of foods, including the eggs and flesh of other animals. Before a year is up, human children can digest a vast array of foodstuffs, virtually the same as an adult. However, no other single foodstuff is as nutritionally complete as milk, which ideally should continue to be the mainstay of the first few years of life.

There are 4,000-odd species of mammals, each with its own milk variant. A different ratio of water, fats, proteins etc applies to each species' milk, and research continually reveals numerous elements of milk that are species-specific. Mammals can digest parts of other mammals' milk from birth, but it will be far from optimum. A human cannot thrive on normal cow's milk until about a year after birth.

Formula Milk

Formula milk is usually based on cow's milk, with a great array of added ingredients: vitamins, amino acids, folic acid, and so on, to make the nutritive ratios closer to human milk. It is also subjected to preservative treatments to stop the milk from souring in storage. It's quite a clever manufactured substance. Whereas normal pasteurised cow's milk is nutritionally insufficient for newborn babies, modern formula milks can sustain growth in human infants

A Big Chapter About Feeding

from birth. Many babies appear to thrive and show no major ill-effects on formula, especially if care is taken to keep the water and feeding equipment sterile, whereas they would become malnourished and sickly on normal cow's milk.

However, formula cow's milk is far from a convincing replica of human milk. Some of the ratios are different, such as more curds than soft whey, which puts a strain on the newborn baby's intestines and kidneys. Unlike with human milk, its consistency does not adjust to thirst, so you may have to supplement it with water. Formula contains some substances not found in human milk, which can trigger allergies. Perhaps most significantly, formula totally lacks the living cells with which human mothers pass on immune defences.

Advantages of Human Milk

Human breastmilk is constantly changing. Just about everything that circulates around your body leaves a trace in it. Your baby will get a milky taste of all that you ingest. This is a good thing, laying the foundation for a receptiveness to a wide range of foodstuffs later. The mammary glands are effective filters, letting through beneficial nutrients, antibodies, macrophages, hormones, enzymes and good bacteria, while minimising potentially harmful substances such as synthetic chemicals, bad bacteria, fungi and viruses. All this is in marked contrast to homogeneous, bland, malty-tasting formula.

Comparative studies consistently show formula-fed babies to be many times more susceptible to allergies, stomach upsets and middle-ear infections, to name a few. This is not to say that all formula-fed babies will frequently be ill (nor that breastfed babies will never be ill), but the likelihood increases.

The benefits of human milk are at their peak in the earliest weeks after birth, when a delicate baby has just entered a world full of infectious agents. Even colostrum (see p114) has a concentration of human-specific nutrients and immunity boosters that will go some way to helping an infant cope with the constant invisible bombardment of viruses and the like. In the first few months of life, when a baby's digestive system is still immature, human milk is by far the easiest food to absorb.

From about six to twelve months, a baby's digestive system matures rapidly and becomes capable of absorbing all manner of things not possible at birth. However, the immune system does not mature until five years of age, thus breastfeeding is still beneficial beyond a year.

For a baby, there are great advantages of breastmilk over formula. Evolution has been less kind to the adult human female, however. Discomfort, maddeningly frequent feeds and social pressures often seem to turn the dispensing of milk into a burden that's hard to bear.

BREASTFEEDING POLITICS

Breastfeeding is the most politicised aspect of babycare. It touches on health, wellbeing and emotional development. It is also tied up with social attitudes and the mores that have formed our own sense of what is natural, what is beneficial and, essentially, what we feel comfortable with.

BREASTFEEDING STATISTICS

Human milk is undoubtedly better than formula milk. The long-term health benefits for babies are summarized in all the up-to-date official literature about babycare, including in this book (see previous pages). In Britain, health officials are obliged to encourage you to breastfeed unless medical conditions in you or your child preclude it (such as chemotherapy). Mothers-to-be who learn about the health benefits of their milk are usually inspired and intent on breastfeeding. Classes are offered by the National Health Service and National Childbirth Trust (NCT). Midwives, health visitors and breastfeeding counsellors who have been trained by the NCT, La Leche League and the Breastfeeding Network are among those who can offer information and support to help you to feed your baby in this way. There is more about these organizations on pp130–131.

Given all this education, encouragement and support, it is astonishing to look at the statistics (left), which show that the majority of women have stopped breastfeeding by six weeks. Mothers generally take the wellbeing of their children to heart, so the switch to bottles with such alacrity suggests a number of adverse factors at work.

Firstly, social context inhibits a widespread continuation of breastfeeding, and there is still a lot of ignorance about the benefits of breastmilk over formula. Breakdowns of the breastfeeding statistics show that age, education and socio-economic status play a part, with the highest level of breastfeeding amongst well-educated women over 30, in social classes I and II, and living in southern England. However, the initial figures released from the latest survey do show an increase in breastfeeding among women who are categorised in lower socio-economic groups. Percentages in virtually all categories have slowly climbed since 1985. The physiological aspects of successful breastfeeding are often not fully understood, resulting in pain and dropping supply (see statistics on p128).

BREASTFEEDING STATISTICS
The percentages of babies being breastfed at different ages:

At birth	67%
1 week	56%
2 weeks	53%
6 weeks	42%
4 months	27%
6 months	21%
9 months	14%

Figures are from the 1995 report of the Office for National Statistics. Exclusive breastfeeding rates are not recorded – the figures include babies who are on a mix of breastmilk and formula.

Figures currently available from the 2000 Infant Feeding Survey show that initial breastfeeding has climbed to 70% in England and Wales, 63% in Scotland and 54% in Northern Ireland.

Some women have an adverse emotional response to breastfeeding and do not enjoy this type of bond with their babies. And some women who do enjoy breastfeeding nevertheless find the intensity of exclusive breastfeeding (no formula at all) too much to bear for long.

Formula Versus Breastmilk

Attitudes to breastfeeding today are to some extent influenced by the beliefs and practices of our own parents and even grandparents. Soon after formula was invented in 1867 by Henri Nestlé (who went on to found the Nestlé commerical empire on the back of his breastmilk substitute), it became positively fashionable. Within a few decades the role of the wet nurse for upper middle-class and aristocratic families had disappeared, and it went on to gradually replace breastfeeding in the majority of families over the next century. From the start, formula was actively promoted as a balanced and highly nutritious milk, which to many implied that breastmilk was a lesser meal.

Furthermore, for decades it was widely believed that bottles were more sanitary than breasts, whereas we are now told the complete opposite – bottles harbour germs and must be sterilised, whereas milk taken from the breast is clean. A belief in the superiority of formula feeding persisted up until the 1970s, our mothers' generation. It is not uncommon to hear disapproval from the older generation of our eagerness to breastfeed. This prejudice can be difficult to overcome. Even when faced with research evidence about the health benefits of breastmilk, your own mother or grandmother might justifiably argue that her tender mothering with the best formula milk of the day didn't appear to do you any harm. Indeed, if you have spent most of your life fit, allergy-free and with a high resistance to infections, you might agree.

Another factor loaded against breastfeeding in our mothers' generation was that the demand-and-supply relationship (see p118) was not fully understood. The nail in the coffin for our breastfeeding mothers and grandmothers was the four-hour feeding schedules (see also p80) followed in many maternity hospitals. For many mothers this did not provide enough stimulation to keep increasing the supply (hungry babies would be left crying until it was time to feed, then only allowed to feed for a few minutes on each side). It is now widely acknowledged that once supply starts to drop and bottles of formula are used to satisfy hunger, there can be a vicious circle whereby the supply drops even further and eventually dries up. It seems that any mother of the 1950s or 1960s who breastfed for more than a few weeks was unusual.

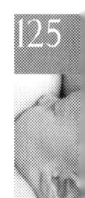

Fortunately, before breastfeeding was abandoned by our culture, scientific research began to reveal all kinds of positive elements in breastmilk. Various pressure groups have successfully campaigned for breastfeeding to be promoted and become more socially accepted. Amongst their successes is a sea-change on many maternity wards, where new mothers are now encouraged to start breastfeeding as soon as possible after delivery. Pressure groups have also managed to limit the overt marketing of formula and bottles. Manufacturers are not allowed to use photographs of babies being bottle-fed on their packaging, nor are they supposed to offer free samples. Because of this renewed focus on breastfeeding, statistics have been steadily climbing since 1980.

In Western culture, however, bottle feeding remains a pervading image. Whilst pictures of naked breasts are commonplace in the media, depictions of breastfeeding are extremely rare. The majority of film or television dramas will opt for a scene of bottle feeding rather than attempt to simulate breastfeeding. The icon of a bottle is often used for babycare facilities and birth congratulation cards; toy dolls sometimes come with bottles.

Breastfeeding in Public

Publicly exposing our breasts – even to the limited extent that feeding necessitates – is not something many of us are used to doing. There are notable exceptions perhaps, such as on warm beaches in sunny climes, but there are many public situations (restaurants, stations, on buses etc) in which you may still face a ripple of unease or even indignation if you were to breastfeed. This has an obvious detrimental effect on the practice, forcing each of us to set self-imposed limits on where we breastfeed. Imagine, if you will, a sliding scale, ranging from doing it only in private at one end to perhaps breastfeeding in the workplace at the other, via way of situations such as family get-togethers, at the park and on public transport. Some women will find themselves more comfortable closer to one end of the scale, others will be just as happy at the other end. Some mothers (and many people more generally) regard nursing a baby as an intensely intimate act, and much prefer for it to be done in private. Others like to pioneer the way with public breastfeeding, and may even confront anyone showing an intolerance of it. And then, of course, there are many who, whilst endorsing the right of women to breastfeed in public places, nevertheless shy away from doing it themselves.

Body Image

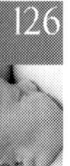

Breasts are an essential part of the feminine image. When you start using them to feed your child your self-image will alter. A lot of women take delight in their new role and feel more womanly. But for some, the sexual focus of breasts is at odds with breastfeeding and wins out over it. Women of the former group are looking at their enlarged, milk-laden breasts and seeing them as voluptuous and nourishing. Women of the latter group may find much about breastfeeding disgusting and a turn-off – some will never start or give up breastfeeding quite soon, whilst others may continue for the sake of the child's health but never actually enjoy it. Size can play a part in this: small-breasted women often like the larger bust, and miss it once they stop breastfeeding; large-breasted women might feel almost handicapped by the extra girth. The attitude from husbands and boyfriends can also have a huge effect.

The breasts change after you've had a child, whether you breastfeed or not. The nipples will probably always be darker; there may be some stretchmarks; and they may sag a bit more (well-fitting breastfeeding bras should minimise sagging). A small minority of women resist breastfeeding in the hope that the bosoms will go back to their former glory.

New Pressures on Women

The politics of breastfeeding do not stop at statistics and social conditioning, however. Partly because the statistics are stacked against them, health authorities and pressure groups tend to proselytise breastfeeding rather than simply recommending it. As a consequence, there is an implied disapproval of mothers who do not breastfeed. Midwives and health visitors are amongst those who might voice dismay to any mother who tries to bottle-feed in the early days.

This disapproval may roll off the back of a mother who has no intention to breastfeed and who is not persuaded that the health benefits to the child are significant. However, a mother who wants to breastfeed, but finds it difficult in practice, may have a miserable time. Many of us develop a mindset that we must soldier on with breastfeeding, even if we are finding it to be a painful and debilitating experience. It's for the good of the child, and, after all, we faced the ordeal of childbirth, so why not this? Alternatively, we feel like failures if we give up before some pre-ordained time, such as at one, three or six months.

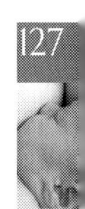

In the early weeks after birth, when we are at our most vulnerable, a sense of failure like this can be profound. For many, breastfeeding is not just about nutrition, it also represents the greatest bond between mother and child, the ultimate maternal ideal. There is another mindset that an inability to nurture your own child through the act of breastfeeding is tantamount to being an "unnatural mother". This idea is reinforced by breastfeeding literature and class leaders who might emphasise the natural aspects of breastfeeding and imply that breastfeeding is essential for bonding. Yet there are many ways of bonding with a child: no-one should imagine that bottle-feeding equates with a lack of care or love. Having spoken to dozens of women on the subject, the editor of this book has no doubt that sometimes breastfeeding can actually get in the way of bonding, especially if emotional difficulties are compounded by pain.

Other breastfeeding women can inadvertently heap the pressure on those who are finding it hard-going. There is a certain competitiveness about motherhood – who sacrifices the most, who is going to breastfeed the longest, who can juggle a career as well, and so on. Women who quickly get into the swing of breastfeeding may not understand the difficulties some others may be facing with pain, or an adverse emotional response, or with a baby being miserable on the breast or, conversely, never wanting to leave it. Remarks like "I'm really proud not to have used a single bottle of formula in four months" are innocently made to other mothers, but can belie this incomprehension.

In a lot of the proselytising literature promoting breastfeeding is an assumption that women who bottle-feed must either be bowing to social prejudice against breastfeeding or not being dedicated enough. There is a lot of advice regarding specific problems such as cracked nipples and mastitis, and encouragements to continue breastfeeding in the face of such problems. With the oft-used maxim "feed on demand", we are given little practical guidance if we find the demands hard to meet (see p134). It can all contribute to postnatal depression.

How Long to Breastfeed?

Whatever your experience of breastfeeding turns out to be, you will stop doing it at some stage, and you are unlikely to be able or want to predict this in advance. Some babies wean themselves, showing less and less interest in the breast. At present, the World Health Organisation, UNICEF and the American Academy of Pediatrics recommend exclusive breastfeeding for six months, and they also point out the health benefits of breastfeeding up to several years of age. The UK Health Authority's *Birth to Five* manual recommends breastfeeding for a year (it doesn't specify whether this should be exclusive). In most babycare manuals you are also told that it's fine if you want to continue breastfeeding beyond a year – there are undoubtedly many health benefits.

Only about one in five women gets to six months with breastfeeding, whether exclusively or partially, and an even smaller minority of mothers breastfeed for a year or more. Those who give up in the first week or two do so because they have had physical or emotional problems with breastfeeding. Many more give up within three to six weeks, often from a worry about supply or ongoing discomfort. Three months is a milestone for many. The onset of weaning onto solids at four to six months is another. The end of maternity leave might be a more obvious marker, however. Another might be when the baby experiments with newly grown front teeth, or becomes easily distracted from

---

REASONS FOR GIVING UP BEFORE SIX WEEKS
A survey was conducted to see why most women have given up breastfeeding by six weeks. The main reasons given were:

- "Insufficient milk"/ baby hungry   48%
- Pain   25%
- Baby would not suck   21%
- Breastfeeding took too long   16%
- Illness (mother or baby)   18%
- Returning to work   2%
- Other   32%

Figures are from the Office for National Statistics. Percentages do not add up to 100 as some mothers gave more than one reason.

A Big Chapter About Feeding

the breast, though some women are not bothered by such things. Yet none of these is an officially sanctioned reason for stopping.

Peer group influence is another factor. This isn't necessarily a pressure, but we commonly compare our own behaviour with other mothers, checking to see if our way of doing things seems reasonable. Hearing of someone else who has started supplementing with bottles at a certain age can make us question ourselves. To be the only one breastfeeding months after everyone else you know has stopped might make you feel the need to actually justify why you are continuing, even though so much official advice is with you. Making contact with one of the breastfeeding support networks can help if this is the case.

Given that one year is the UK recommendation for breastfeeding and also the age when a child can go on to normal cow's milk rather than formula, it is an obvious goal for mothers who breastfeed exclusively or partially beyond six months. On the other hand, there are still immunological benefits of breastmilk for many years. It is also possible to practice "tandem feeding" of a toddler and young baby at the same time. Yet mothers who continue to breastfeed beyond a year might do so in the face of astonishment from those who stopped long before. Astonishment can rapidly turn to disapproval, however, and there is huge prejudice against mothers who continue to breastfeed into the third year, the fourth and beyond. In the US there have even been some charges of sexual abuse in cases of prolonged breastfeeding. Basically, whatever stage a mother stops breastfeeding winds up being a socially charged message to others.

Breastfeeding in Other Cultures

In developing nations, breastfed babies have a much greater chance of survival than those who are bottle-fed with formula – not only does formula lack the immune system boosters to help infants fight disease, but the water used to mix with formula may be dirty, and the bottle-feeding equipment hard to sterilize, leading to often lethal illnesses. Nestlé has been villified for promoting its infant formula milk in developing nations. The International Baby Food Action Network (IBFAN) drew up the 1981 International Code of Marketing of Breastmilk Substitutes (right) and various other provisions that limit the marketing of formula. By 1999, 20 countries had signed up to the code.

Looking at other cultures from another angle, breastfeeding pressure groups often make references to societies in which breastfeeding is the norm in order to promote the practice in our own society. There are a lot of striking contrasts: the Western world has an astonishingly repressive attitude towards breastfeeding when compared with societies in which it is done openly without prejudice. In order to illustrate points about social conditioning, the pressure

CODE FOR MARKETING FORMULA
The International Code of Marketing of Breastmilk Substitutes states:

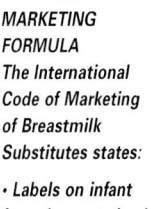

• Labels on infant formula must clearly state the superiority of breastfeeding, include preparation instructions and a warning about the health hazards of inappropriate preparation.

• There should be no pictures of infants or other pictures or text idealising the use of infant formula on labels. The terms "humanised", "maternalised" or similar should not be used.

• Labels of all products under the Code should provide the necessary information about the appropriate use of the product and should be designed so as not to discourage breastfeeding.

(Annual sales of baby milk are worth about US$8 billion.)

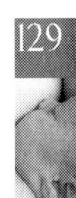

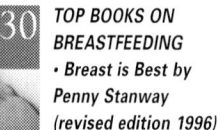

TOP BOOKS ON
BREASTFEEDING
• Breast is Best by
Penny Stanway
(revised edition 1996)

• Breastfeeding Your
Baby by Heather
Welford (Marshall
Editions, 2000)

• The Womanly Art
of Breastfeeding by
Gwen Gotsch for La
Leche League (Plume
Books 1997)

• The National
Childbirth Trust Book
of Breastfeeding,
Mary Smale (1999)

• Bestfeeding
(Renfrew, Fisher and
Arms, 2000)

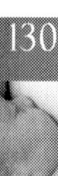

groups have gone so far as to cite examples of societies in which seven-year-old children are breastfed and grandmothers breastfeed their grandchildren. But few people in Western society seriously want to emulate such practices, thus breastfeeding continues to be a culturally sensitive area.

BREASTFEEDING SUPPORT

As mentioned earlier, midwives and health visitors can help to encourage and sort out any problems with breastfeeding. Unfortunately, due to the midwife shortage, there is not always that much time for them to discuss queries in detail. The level of support they can provide may depend on their individual breadth of experience in the field. Some midwives and health visitors are mothers, but others will not have experienced breastfeeding for themselves.

There are a number of other sources if you are experiencing difficulty with breastfeeding, not least the many books devoted to the subject (left). The groups listed below disseminate information about the benefits and best techniques of breastfeeding. They also provide a breastfeeding "community" that can be of immense value to women who want to breastfeed but do not feel well supported by society at large.

It is important to understand that such pressure groups and support networks are run by people (mainly mothers) who care passionately about encouraging a more widespread acceptance of breastfeeding in our society as well as a desire to help fellow mothers through any difficulties with breastfeeding. They are highly knowledgeable about breastfeeding but not necessarily other areas of health, as are midwives and health visitors. One criticism that has been levelled at such organisations is that the way in which they disseminate information about the benefits of breastfeeding does not allow for any "excuse" not to breastfeed, even if a woman is experiencing physical and emotional difficulties with it. Therefore, they have been accused of creating undue pressure on women to breastfeed.

La Leche League International (LLL) Pronounced la-lay-shay, this organisation was founded in the USA in 1956 by seven mothers and others concerned that the percentage of American women breastfeeding had dropped to 20%. In their own words, their mission "is to help mothers worldwide to breastfeed through mother-to-mother support, encouragement, information and education, and to promote a better understanding of breastfeeding as an important element in the healthy development of the baby and the mother." Recognised by UNICEF and the WHO, the campaigning of La Leche over the years has helped to more than treble breastfeeding statistics. UK phone 020 7242 1278. www.laleche.org.uk

NCT Breastfeeding Counsellors The UK's National Childbirth Trust has long been involved with the promotion of breastfeeding in this country and has trained several hundred volunteers as breastfeeding counsellors – see Heather Welford's statement about their services below. If you want to be put in touch with a local counsellor, phone 0870 333 1487. The service is free.

The Breastfeeding Network (BFN) The founders of this were former NCT breastfeeding counsellors who felt compromised by the NCT's decision to accept sponsorship from a formula manufacturer. The support number is 0870 900 8787; www.breastfeeding.co.uk/bfn

Baby Milk Action A British pressure group that works with IBFAN to campaign against companies that have not signed to or violate the International Code of Marketing of Breastmilk Substitutes. www.babymilkaction.org

Views From Two Experts
A statement by Heather Welford about the services offered by NCT breastfeeding counsellors

"NCT breastfeeding counsellors don't see themselves as offering advice to mothers. We offer support and information, and we use counselling techniques to enable a mother to decide for herself how she deals with or resolves concerns about infant feeding. Some of the information might include the health effects of feeding choices, and techniques to enable breastfeeding to be effective and pain-free.

We recognise that many women stop breastfeeding before they planned to, and that parents' rights to exercise choice and make fully informed decision-making about infant feeding may be affected by complex social, individual and cultural factors.

We campaign for the right of mothers to breastfeed and to do so where they wish, for as long as they wish. We campaign for better edcation and training among health professionals, in schools and in society as a whole, and for improved employment conditions and flexible provision for leave, and for continuing to breastfeed while in paid employment. We make a distinction between campaigning, and supporting women on an individual basis. In practice, breastfeeding counsellors discuss formula feeding with mothers, and the use of bottles, and we recognise that breastfeeding is more than just a way of getting a healthy food and drink into babies – mothers may have a complex agenda, and need the chance to talk it through with someone who will not judge them. All NCT events are open and welcoming to parents, no matter how they are feeding, and should be publicised as such. Our Baby Feeding Policy outlines our approach." (See phone number and website on previous page.)

A statement about breastfeeding politics
by babycare writer Robin Barker (see p81)

"It is indisputable that a solid body of scientific evidence is now available showing that breastfeeding has advantages that cannot be matched by infant formula. It is also indisputable that there are still significant numbers of women who do not breastfeed because of a lack of information, their economic and educational status and inaccurate advice from health professionals when problems arise.

There is, however, a growing band of women who are fully informed about all aspects of breastfeeding and who have access to dedicated health professionals who give accurate advice. A number of these women are devastated when, despite everyone's best efforts, their breastfeeding doesn't work out as they expect it to. Problems that lead to breastfeeding being abandoned in the first six weeks include clinical problems that never get resolved and unexpected social and psychological factors.

After 20 years of talking to women about breastfeeding and helping new mothers to do it, I firmly believe that, as breastfeeding success cannot be guaranteed for every woman, pregnant women should be prepared for every possible outcome. It should be remembered that, with the best will in the world, about two women in ten will experience breastfeeding problems that cannot be resolved. And that, for others, a superhuman effort might be required to maintain breastfeeding until time (up to three months) brings rewards which understandably might be beyond some women.

I am aware my view particularly as a health professional in the field might be seen as negative, even counter-productive in the interests of getting everyone to breastfeed. I firmly believe, however, too many women today are being pushed beyond endurance during the first three months with complicated breastfeeding regimes that do not work, and are then left feeling inadequate and hopeless, even bereft when the breastfeeding doesn't work out. More often than not the breastfeeding professional mutters a few words of sympathy before disappearing, leaving the mother alone trying to make sense of it all.

It is not my intention to dissuade women from taking the best option. Rather it is a call to health professionals and those involved in the promotion, protection and support of breastfeeding to give first-time mothers a greater understanding of the reality of breastfeeding and the possible problems that may make breastfeeding a greater challenge than they anticipate."

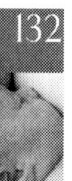

A Big Chapter About Feeding

VIEWS FROM MOTHERS

Many women interviewed for the book had strong opinions about the way in which breastfeeding is promoted. Emma T. had already become highly aware of the politics by the time she was seven months pregnant. "All the stuff that's written about breastfeeding talks about the benefits, whereas all the mothers I know talk about the problems," she said.

Jane S. had been breastfeeding for two weeks when asked for her views. "Breastfeeding is going quite well, though it is rather painful and no-one warned me that I would be doing it for about six hours each day! Also, I get a bit depressed with all the leaking at night and the baby's posset all over my clothes. As for the politics, there was a woman on my postnatal ward who asked a midwife for a bottle of formula because she had a bad experience breastfeeding her first baby. Three midwives then came and lectured her for ages about the benefits of breastfeeding, but she kept saying "I understand all that, now please get me a bottle". I was amazed at both the mother and the way in which she was being pressurised."

Nicky's belief is that "if you have brought a child into this world then you have an obligation to breastfeed, the same as you have an obligation to give up smoking, for the sake of your child's health. Yes, it can be painful – I was biting on wood with the pain – but you can get through that."

Dawn also had a forthright view, from the opposite corner. "I get angry when I hear people saying how breastfeeding is natural, easy and beneficial for both mother and baby. It may be "natural" in the biological sense, but then so are mastitis or dying in childbirth! The information about breastfeeding just tells you about the health benefits and how to deal with engorgement and problems, but there is an emotional side too. I think that there is far too much fuss over breastfeeding, as if your baby will suffer for life if you bottle-feed. I can't empathise with women who make a big show of expressing their milk when they go back to work – being there in person for your child is more important than whether you choose to breastfeed or not."

Kirstie thought that the breastfeeding workshops should make it clearer that full breastfeeding is a tremendous task – "the mother gets no time off day or night for many months, and it takes responsibility away from the father, too". However, Amy, a supporter of Baby Milk Action, says that there should be more focus on the positive aspects of breastfeeding. "Most mothers give up because they don't understand technique. If it wasn't for groups like BMA, no-one would be breastfeeding anymore. As it is, about one in three women never starts, and hospital practice often works against breastfeeding." Amy was the only mother interviewed who did not think we are under much pressure to breastfeed.

FEEDING RHYTHMS

Questions about how long feeds should go on for, what kind of feeding pattern you might get into, and how to cope with night feeds might start to preoccupy your mind soon after you begin the task of breastfeeding. There's little concensus about such matters. Finding ways that work for both you and your baby will be important over the coming months.

A CLOSER LOOK AT FEEDING ON DEMAND

"Feed on demand" is a common piece of advice. In other words, just feed your baby whenever he or she wants to feed, not according to a pre-ordained schedule. Among the reasons for this recommendation is because the majority of babies are capable of regulating their own intake of milk to suit their changing needs. If they are hungrier than normal, they will feed more frequently, and your supply will be automatically boosted to match demand (see p118).

Following a simple policy of feeding on demand works well for a lot of women, whose babies will thrive on it. But it does not work for everyone, especially not for women who are having difficulties with breastfeeding, or who are in a state of exhaustion. The advice is controversial, though relatively few new mothers are aware of the controversy at first. "Feed on demand" is probably best viewed as a simplistic catch-phrase for a general policy, not the solution for every situation.

Criticism of demand feeding is angled from several levels. For a start, thinking in terms of "demands" sets the baby up as a bit of a tyrant. Some experts prefer the terms "request feeding" or "response feeding" to get away from this kind of negative connotation.

Then how is the "demand" or "request" going to be made? Through crying. A hunger cry is of course hard to distinguish from any other kind of cry in a newborn (see the crying checklist on p93). In some ways, whether it really is a hunger cry or not doesn't matter. What many mothers find is that their newborn baby will nearly always stop crying when offered the breast – it provides food and comfort, both of which babies crave. In fact, offering a feed every time your newborn starts crying is probably a reasonable policy for many new mothers whilst breastfeeding is being established. Indeed, a lot of mothers are genuinely happy to continue in this vein for many weeks to come, finding it the most obvious and easiest way to gain peace and bonding with the baby. On the other hand, it is not essential to answer every kind of cry with a feed, especially not if you are finding frequent breastfeeding painful and debilitating. The catch-phrase "feed on demand" is inadequate for situations like these.

It's easy to see how "feed on demand" can be taken too literally. New mothers soon begin to anticipate their own babies' needs. In fact, most people would agree that there's no need ever to wait for a demand before offering a feed. Being able to pre-empt at least some of the crying will be a way in which you'll build confidence in your skills as a parent.

Perhaps the worst way in which "feed on demand" can be taken too literally is with sleepy babies who rarely cry and can become dehydrated through inadequate milk intake. Usually, paediatricians spot these babies – they may be sleepy if certain drugs were used during labour – and will probably recommend that you wake the baby up to feed at certain intervals. Other worrying scenarios might be if the latching-on isn't right (see pp115–116), so that the baby doesn't get all the milk in your breasts, or if your milk supply drops considerably, so that even with very frequent demand feeding your baby is still not getting enough food, and you are becoming stressed (see pp139–141).

Demand Feeding Versus a Feeding Schedule

In much of today's popular babycare literature is a demonisation of feeding schedules. This attitude arose when the strict babycare regimes of the mid-20th century were challenged by the post-War baby-centred approach (see p85). Moreover, the four-hour feeding regimes followed in many maternity wards up to the 1970s were proven to be counter-productive in establishing breastfeeding. To leave a four-hour gap between feeds, then only feed for a few minutes on each side, does not provide enough stimulation to keep up the milk supply in the majority of women, and thus few babies are happy about it either. With the big swing to the baby-centred approach, one of the main concepts was never to impose any time constraints on feeding.

A minority of today's popular babycare writers, including "routine queen" Gina Ford, and sleep experts such as Richard Ferber, say that instigating a routine is best, and that the baby will soon get used to being fed at specific times (as well as being put to bed at specific times). Some people are adamant that having a 24-hour structure can be of immense psychological and physiological benefit to parent and child.

The counter-argument from those who advise demand feeding is that all babies are different and it is unfair to expect all of them to conform to a routine, and the only way you can be sure that the baby is getting enough to eat is if you feed on demand. If you let the baby lead the way, some kind of a feeding and sleeping pattern will eventually emerge.

Thus, in babycare literature today, it often seems like an either/or choice – you either follow a regime or you always wait for your baby to demand food. Only a few of the experts suggest that there is a middle ground. Despite this, the middle ground is frequently traversed by mothers themselves. Many start out by feeding on demand, then, as breastfeeding becomes established, try to encourage a feeding pattern that will dovetail with a sleep pattern – thus finding a rough routine that works for their individual circumstances. This is looked at more closely later in this chapter.

Some Views About Demand Feeding

Justine happily breastfed on demand for six months: "Feeding on demand worked out fairly well. I think that sometimes I fed her when she wasn't really hungry, but I wanted a rest and a cuddle anyway. I was very surprised at the frequency of feeds in the early days. As Ella got older, and her stomach bigger, frequency and urgency decreased. Breastfeeding on demand does mean you have your bosoms out a lot, but that didn't worry me."

Emma: "I don't like the idea of on-demand feeding at all – you spend all day doing it, and from what I've heard it takes far longer for your child to sleep through the night."

Annette: "I think demand feeding is fine once you have grown to know your baby over a few weeks. In the early days it can be confusing, as there's a tendency to think that every time the baby cries she is hungry, which is not always the case."

Kelly: "The advice about feeding was confusing. The paediatrician said wait two hours between feeds to give my nipples a rest, one of the midwives said wake my baby to feed every three hours because she's small, and another one said feed whenever she cries. I didn't have the energy to figure it all out, and never had a proper strategy. Sometimes I would feed her because more than three hours had passed, and sometimes she insisted on snacking every hour, though I might try and put her off until two hours had gone by. I was so tired all the time, but somehow got through to three months with the breastfeeding."

Amy: "Feeding on demand is definitely the best approach. Babies love it, and you have peace of mind knowing that this is the best foundation for their health and attachment to you. You also get to rest a lot – no-one expects you to rush around with a baby latched on. I still breastfeed my one-year-old on demand several times a day and when he wakes up at night."

Ellie: "I fed on demand for a month, but he didn't get into a pattern on his own, just wanted to feed the whole time. Then I started on Gina Ford because I craved a routine – I wanted to have that feeling of "mother knows best". He took to the routine really well, going from about 12 or more little feeds down to 7 big ones in the space of three days. I thought some of her timings were too strict, however, and adapted them. At postnatal yoga, I was the only one not getting my boobs out twice an hour. Perhaps the others thought they were bonding better with their babies, but to me it looked like they just wanted to shut them up if they made any sort of noise. Five months on, I am still breastfeeding, which is a lot longer than some of the demand feeders lasted."

Length of Feeds

How long each individual feed should last is also subject to differing opinions. A few decades ago, mothers were told to feed for five or ten minutes each side, but this notion is almost universally rejected nowadays. Few newborn babies are adept enough to get to the hindmilk in five or even ten minutes, though they may become capable of this as they grow older. Some lactation experts say that 20 to 30 minutes is more likely for a young baby, and sometimes even longer. Babies do vary in their sucking capabilities, and positioning (see pp115–116) can also affect the length of feeds. Basically, every baby and every feed are different, so some breastfeeding counsellors say it is better to look at the pattern of the feed (see the next section) rather than think in terms of minutes.

The usual advice now is to let your baby feed on one breast until he either comes away from the breast or falls asleep. If he comes away, you can try offering the other breast to see if he is still hungry. Letting your baby suck for as long as he wants is part of the broad "feed on demand" advice – it works well while breastfeeding is being established, and some women are happy to continue with it indefinitely. But it doesn't have to apply to all situations. An important factor to consider is that many babies will continue sucking for sheer pleasure after they have imbibed all the milk they need and there is little left in your breast. This does not have to be a problem, especially not if you love breastfeeding and find it peaceful. Comfort sucking can also induce sleep in your baby, which you might be longing for. On the other hand, feeding-to-sleep can be a problematic part of sleep conditioning as the weeks go by (see pp176–177), and you wouldn't be the only mother to sometimes feel frustrated, glued to the chair waiting for your child to finish. Some women work out a way of using a sling so that the baby can feed while they move around.

Feeding Rhythms

If You Want to Limit Comfort Sucking

How to tell when the baby has fed enough and is continuing just for pleasure? If your baby is latched on well and ready for a full feed, typically you might find that at first the sucking is strong and fairly continuous for many minutes (don't count the moments when your baby pauses to swallow). After a while – a very rough guideline would be 10 or 20 minutes – the pace will start to slow. Your baby is perhaps on the hindmilk by this stage. One NCT breastfeeding counsellor describes a kind of "fluttering" suck once the hindmilk has been finished. Note that there will always be a tiny bit of foremilk left in your breast. After this, the sucking might become intermittent, stopping for long seconds, then perhaps starting up again for a while when you move or stroke the baby's cheek. This final intermittent kind of sucking is thus more likely to be for comfort than sustenance. (But see also the section on Snacking below.)

If you think your baby has fed enough and you want to limit comfort sucking, you could try unlatching (use a finger to break suction) and see what the reaction is. There may be a protest for a few seconds, in which case you could try distracting the baby's attention or place him in his bed for a nap, if he is due for one. Many people use dummies, though their prolonged use can be problematic (see p100). If your baby still seems hungry then offer the other breast if you haven't already and see if the sucking goes full force again. You will get to know the pattern of your baby's feeding after a while.

It's up to you if you want to limit comfort sucking on your breast or not. Some people think it's ok to limit it and that dummies and other comforts such as swaddling are a good stand-in, and, eventually finger- and thumb-sucking will be the comfort (once the baby has worked out how to control the hands, from about four months). On the other hand, there is a school of thought that after-dinner pleasure sucking on the breast is all part of an essential bonding process for both mother and child, so you should never curtail it. Indeed, a lot of the pro-breastfeeding literature carries through an underlying assumption that breastfeeding is one of the most essential elements of bonding. (The editor of this book does not agree with that view – see also pp127 and 211.)

Babies Who Seem to Snack

If you do not recognise the description of a full feed described above, and your baby only ever spends a few minutes on the breast, before dozing off, coming off or fussing, and feeds more frequently than, say, 12 times in 24 hours, then he may be snacking rather than taking full, breast-emptying feeds. It seems that some babies snack from birth, sometimes perhaps because they haven't developed a good latch. Others might develop the habit as the weeks go by as

A Big Chapter About Feeding

a side-effect of being offered feeds when they are not particularly hungry. Again, it's not necessarily a problem, only if you perceive it as such. If your baby normally takes full feeds but goes through a patch of snacking, this is not necessarily anything to worry about – maybe it's a hot day and he needs extra drinks. Look at the pattern over a whole week, not just the last two days.

Then again, some babies perpetually want to snack for a few minutes almost every hour (even several times an hour), and only sleep in short bursts of an hour or two, day after day. It's hardly surprising that this kind of exhausting scenario is often cited as a reason for switching to formula. If the frequency of the snacking is making you despair with breastfeeding, it might be worth seeing if you can lengthen the feeds and bring the feeding frequency down to a manageable level before resorting to formula (assuming you would otherwise be happy about breastfeeding). What consitutes "manageable" obviously depends on the baby and how much energy you have, but the minimum is going to be six or eight feeds in 24 hours for a newborn, or roughly every three or four hours (i.e. the same frequency as for bottle-feeding a newborn).

If you are trying to get away from hourly or half-hourly feeding, it's probably best not to try and leap to a three-hourly schedule in one go. A better way to go about it might be to put off feeding your baby for increasing intervals of, say, 15 minutes at a time. Unfortunately, you will probably have to listen to crying because your baby will literally be hungry, having got used to snacking. However, what you will be looking out for is that the feed will be longer when it does happen, and that it will hopefully get down to the hindmilk in your breasts in one go, and that any hunger crying will become shorter in duration with each feed.

It can get so confusing with frequent snacking that you don't know what constitutes a single feed – maybe the baby goes on and off the breast four or five times in an hour, then sleeps for two hours, then snacks on and off for another two hours, and so on. A health visitor or breastfeeding counsellor may be able to discuss your individual circumstances and suggest ways of getting through without you having to turn to formula in desperation. Ultimately, your personal feelings about breastfeeding will dictate the course of action.

Not Having Enough Milk

Not having enough milk is the number one reason cited by women who start supplementing with formula or give up breastfeeding altogether. The scenario can be similar to that described under snacking. However, rather than leaving you with milk to spare, the feeding takes all the milk from both breasts, and before long, perhaps in the space of an hour, the baby seriously wants to feed again, before your breasts have had much chance to produce more milk.

Feeding Rhythms

Supply always fluctuates according to demand (see p118), and your breasts get the signal to pump up the volume when they are emptied and the frequency of feeds increases. The extra volume may take a few days to appear, but if breastfeeding is already established and in a good rhythm – a full feed every few hours – you are unlikely to experience a huge drop in supply even during times of the so-called growth spurts, when babies become more hungry than usual for a few days at a time. It is if more than a few days go by with low supply that the problems become pronounced.

When breastfeeding is hard to establish in the first place – such as when the latch isn't good, or there have been infrequent feeds in the first few days – a vicious circle can appear of dwindling supply and supplementation with formula. This (and pain with latching-on) is why many unfortunate women never get beyond the first week of breastfeeding. Stress itself can inhibit the let-down of milk, another element in the circle.

It is often possible to boost very low supply with very frequent feeding and bed-rest to minimise stress. Unfortunately, it doesn't always work, especially if breastfeeding was never established in the first place and the mother is already exhausted and unhappy. Worse still, mothers do not always get the sympathy and support they need in such difficult circumstances. Consider Sally's story:

Sally wanted to breastfeed but had problems right from the start: "The days following birth were very stressful because the baby had jaundice, and I was exhausted. I think it was because of this early stress that my body never produced enough milk. In the first weeks, Thomas would feed for at least an hour at a time and yet still be hungry. He appeared to be sucking properly, so I didn't think there was a problem with positioning. But nothing helped to boost my supply. One awful afternoon, I was stuck on the sofa for five hours while he continually fed and fed, shrieking whenever I tried to stop him and get up.

I was so shattered by the situation that I didn't know what to do or say to anyone. My husband was the one who phoned a breastfeeding counsellor. She suggested that I end a feed after 40 minutes and try to divert Thomas's attention with games or taking him for a walk – maybe he was a very "sucky" baby, doing it for comfort. We tried this, but he would scream throughout the whole walk until I fed him again. Despite all the feeding, my supply seemed to be dropping, not increasing. Hardly anything came out when I expressed either. What swung it in the end was that he wasn't gaining the expected weight and we had tried everything the breastfeeding counsellor suggested. So we took our own decision to let him feed from me for up to an hour at a time, then give him a bottle of formula as a top-up. To our relief he stopped crying so much.

I still wanted to breastfeed, but he soon lost interest because he knew that a bottle was coming. I consulted two health visitors, but didn't get much help: one didn't mind me mixing breast and bottles and seemed to think it inevitable that I would soon switch fully to formula; the other said that we should know we were exposing Thomas to a greater risk of cot death by feeding him formula. This was deeply upsetting to hear, as you can imagine. I continued with a mix of breast and bottles for some weeks in total misery. He was mainly happy with the bottles, though, and I eventually gave up breastfeeding at about three months.

I have thought a lot about how the situation developed, and with my next child I intend to rest more in the early days – my husband will have to do absolutely everything else while I lie in bed with the new baby..."

The situation of having a very low supply and a hungry baby can be horrible. If you find yourself in this situation or think that you might be heading that way, it's worth consulting a midwife, health visitor or breastfeeding counsellor, and getting more opinions if need be, because there are a lot of opinions out there. Unfortunately, much of the popular literature on breastfeeding neglects to mention the possibility of exhaustion in mothers who are feeding very frequently. Worse still, some of the literature, especially on the Internet, equates frequent breastfeeding with worthy self-sacrifice – if you really care about your child's health you will put any thoughts about tiredness or discomfort to one side and feed every half hour or whatever it takes. There is also a certain amount of scare-mongering about what might happen to your baby if you start supplementing, which might leave you with the impression that rather than just being a second-best but reasonable option, formula is an evil, alien substance, and that bottles break the bonding process. A lot of us believe in a certain level of maternal sacrifice. But mothers are not machines – your own state of health and mind is important, too.

Anyhow, leaving this unhappy scenario to one side, it should be reiterated that if you can establish a regular breastfeeding rhythm in the first few weeks, you are unlikely to experience a vast drop in supply.

Establishing Breastfeeding

Unless birth has left you in a really bad way, do try to nurse your newborn within the first couple of hours. Fascinatingly, most newborns have a strong instinct to find the nipple and suck in the first hours of life outside the womb, but if the desire is not met, it is said that the craving can strangely fade for a couple of days, before coming back. The use of drugs in labour can also inhibit the baby's sucking instincts. But don't worry, all is not lost if you are unable to breastfeed

Feeding Rhythms

initially. Even if your baby is given formula or a sugar and water solution for several feeds while you sleep (see p181), you still have every chance to take over with breastfeeding. Just start offering the breast as soon as you can, taking great care with positioning (see the photos on p115). Because of the midwife shortage (see p24), there may not be that much practical help and encouragement with breastfeeding, but it's worth seeking out any advice midwives have to offer in the crucial early days.

If you experience discomfort for more than a few seconds as the milk lets down, check positioning and maybe unlatch and try again to get more areola in. The baby's lower jaw should do the work. Sometimes, everything looks right, but ongoing nipple pain tells you it's not. In the first hectic days after birth, it may be best to try and push virtually all other parts of your life to one side while you and your baby get used to breastfeeding, and immediately seek help with any problems. At first, it may also be best to follow the "feed on demand" policy unless a health professional tells you otherwise, such as if your baby is "sleepy" and needs waking to feed. Frequent feeding – every couple of hours – is the norm at this stage. This sort of frequency is good for establishing breastfeeding, but unfortunately it means that you are not going to get much sleep, at a time when you probably desperately need it. Having someone else stand in with a bottle of expressed milk or formula while you sleep is obviously an option, but something to be wary of when done frequently (see pp147–149).

Once your milk comes in you will hopefully soon get into the swing of feeding. It's often said that breastfeeding takes several weeks to establish, after which you should not be experiencing much, if any, discomfort. You will also be understanding your baby's habits a lot better and able to anticipate feeds as breastfeeding becomes established.

Finding Your Own Feeding Rhythm

As shown before, feeding routines are a controversial area. Some people are adamant that you shouldn't try to apply a routine; others are just as adamant that you can if you want. In support of the former view, if you are happy with the baby-led frequency and duration of breastfeeding, there's certainly no reason to tinker with the situation – you're already in the rhythm that's right for both your baby and you, even if it bears no resemblance to the kind of feeding schedule touted by some experts.

This and the next section are for those who are unhappy with unpredictable, sporadic demand feeding around the clock, with no sign of a rhythm emerging of its own accord. You are desperately tired and feel like abandoning breastfeeding just so you can have some respite from the relentless

TIP: Once breastfeeding is established, you may find that your breasts rarely feel full like they did at first, which might lead you to believe that there's not much milk in them. In fact, you may be producing a lot more milk than in the early days, but your breasts will have adapted. A parallel can be drawn with the way a pair of stiff leather shoes might have to be worn in before they feel comfortable!

babycare. Whatever the motivation, it might help to try to instigate more of a 24-hour rhythm before resorting to formula.

To start with, it's perhaps better to consider the overall number of feeds in 24 hours rather than the timings in between them, because few babies take kindly to a strict routine, and too few feeds could lead to a drop in your milk supply. As a guide, it is generally accepted that young babies need an absolute minimum of six full feeds in 24 hours, whether breast or bottle. Some experts actually state that six to eight full breastfeeds are sufficient. If you find that you are continually feeding on demand a lot more than this, then it may be worth exploring whether this is due to a lot of comfort sucking by your baby, especially if it is becoming a part of sleep conditioning (see p176). Simply bringing the overall number of feeds down might ease distress over breastfeeding without having to apply strict timings. It is often more the baby's sleep times that the mother wants to regulate than the feeding frequency. Encouraging a different frequency between day and night feeds is a popular ploy (see next sections).

With a loose and flexible routine, you tread the middle ground between demand feeding and strict regime, a place that many find is very good to be. There are numerous ways in which you can encourage a loose feeding routine based on your growing knowledge of your baby's habits. Indeed, following the baby's lead on timings, then coaxing them into a 24-hour routine is probably what the majority of mothers end up doing, despite all the literature on the subject exhorting you either not to live by the clock at all or to let it rule every aspect of your parental life. This applies to both feeding and sleep times.

With a loose feeding rhythm, you will be looking to feed at roughly the same times in every 24 hours. This will help circadian rhythms to develop faster (see pp160–161). For example, some babies quickly develop a fairly regular feeding frequency, say, every two-and-a-half or three hours, but through taking an extra long sleep once a day or having odd snacking periods, do not fall into a regular 24-hour, circadian pattern. If this is the case, you could try regulating feeds roughly to the most common frequency and see if this helps the situation. Certainly, if your baby normally feeds about every three hours, but starts crying just an hour after the last feed, it's worth exploring other reasons for the crying, especially the possibility of tiredness, before you offer an interim feed.

Trying to create a 24-hour circadian rhythm might involve waking up your baby specifically to feed now and then – think about feeding in conjunction with a sleep rhythm. Once a basic 24-hour cycle has been established, you may find that you have a certain leeway with timings, or that your baby adopts differing rhythms of feeding in phases. A loose routine is always an amorphous, two-way process between you and your baby.

Feeding Rhythms

Four-hour schedules (six breastfeeds in 24 hours) can work for a minority of women who have no difficulty with milk supply and whose babies perhaps have a greater stomach capacity at birth than most. More frequent feeds, such as a rough three-hour schedule (eight feeds in 24 hours) have a better chance. In Japan, two-and-a-half-hour breastfeeding schedules during daytime are recommended by some doctors.

If you enjoyed a highly structured life before having a baby, you are more likely to appreciate a strict routine. Gina Ford (see p82) offers a strict schedule for a two-week-old baby of seven feeds within 24 hours timed to the minute, at intervals varying from one to four hours. Various feeds are dropped as the months go by, beginning with the night feeds, until there are just three daytime feeds by the age of about six months. Some people rave about her routine, some say it didn't work for them.

Note that the intervals are timed from the start of feeds, because babies vary in how long they take to suck the milk out.

A Feed-Awake-Nap Daytime Rhythm

A pattern that can work well from a young age is a recurring feed-awake-nap rhythm during the day. With this you would offer a full feed as soon as your baby wakes up from a nap (not waiting for a hunger cry). After the feed, you would then encourage your baby to be awake and active for an hour or so. Then you would encourage another nap (see p175). If you want to try out this rhythm, avoid inducing the next nap with another feed if possible, so that your baby does not learn to rely on feeding in order to sleep. Around three hours from the start of the last feed – or two-and-a-half, three-and-a-half or four hours, based on your knowledge of your baby's behaviour – feed your baby again, waking him if necessary. Repeat the feed-awake-nap rhythm three or four times during daytime. You may find that your baby slips quite easily into this rhythm within a matter of days. But don't despair if not.

Many people apply the evening feeding times more strictly and are not so bothered about the timing of daytime feeds (or sleeps) so long as there is a basic division between night and day. Once established, the recurring feed-awake-nap rhythm can remain in place for many months, until your baby is ready to drop the daytime naps one by one.

Night Feeding Rhythms

Eventually, your baby will be capable of getting through the whole night without feeding, and it's worth encouraging this wherever possible (see also the Sleep chapter). One way might be to feed the baby with more frequency during daytime in the hope that there will be automatically less call for night feeds. And whereas in the daytime you might want to feed long before your baby starts crying with hunger, at night wait for the hunger cry. Then again, some people wake their baby specially to feed about an hour before they plan to go to bed, in the hope that they will get a more predictable stretch of sleep and be woken only once in the early hours, rather than two or three times. Penelope Leach is one of the proponents of this kind of night feed juggling.

As babies' sleep capabilities mature, they often start dropping the night feeds of their own accord (see p170), "sleeping through" in progressively longer phases. If this doesn't happen naturally – some babies get used to feeding at night, especially if they are always fed-to-sleep – another thing to try after two or three months is limiting the length of night feeds and eventually not offering them at all. To do this with confidence, you will need to be sure that your baby is taking in lots of food during the daytime. A newborn's stomach does not have the capacity to take in enough food during daytime (it is about the size of a walnut). But many three-month-old babies do have the capacity.

An unfortunate side-effect of your baby taking fewer night feeds is that your breasts may become over-full, leaking and waking you up in the night. To minimise this problem, some women express just before going to bed.

Expressing

Being able to express milk is useful for relieving engorgement, for feeding premature babies who can't suck properly, for helping to boost supply if need be, and for times when you want to do something else for a few hours (go out or just sleep perhaps) while someone else feeds the expressed milk, either from a cup or a bottle.

To hand express, make sure you are warm, comfortable and not in a hurry about anything. Cup your fingers around one breast and squeeze and draw down the areola. Nothing may come out at first, but after a few goes you will hopefully feel the let-down. Carry on with the milking action and the milk should start to flow. If not, try squeezing from a different angle – there are several ducts. Some women find expressing easy, with the milk coming out in amusing sprays. You will need a big bowl if this is the case! And some women are never able to get more than a few drops out. Even if you find it easy, hand expressing can take ages. There are several makes of breastpump on the market, which might speed up expressing. Some are hand-operated; some are powered by batteries; some are powered from the mains. You may be able to express straight into a bottle using a pump. However, if your milk doesn't let down with hand expressing, it may not with a pump either. The electrical pumps are especially expensive

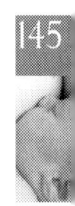

Feeding Rhythms

items, given that most women only want to express occasionally, so borrow one if you can. Sometimes they can be hired.

If you are expressing to create a meal for your baby rather than just to get rid of some excess milk, then everything the milk comes into contact with needs to be sterile (not just clean). That includes the pump itself as well as the receptacles for the milk. There are three main sterilizing methods: boiling for five minutes, which merely requires a large saucepan; leaving to soak in a chemical sterilising solution for several hours (widely available in chemists and supermarkets); or being run through a baby bottle steamer cycle for 10 minutes or so (available in some chemists and babycare shops). It may seem strange to have to sterilize when you don't have to keep your own breasts in a sterile state, but once milk leaves the body it becomes one of the most volatile of foodstuffs, a wonderful culture for bacteria. (Consider how quickly unpasteurised cow's milk goes off.) You will need to store the milk either in the fridge, using it within 24 hours, or in a deep freezer, where it will last up to three months.

Bear in mind that your baby may have no idea how to feed from anything other than your breast. Try introducing some expressed milk from a cup or bottle a few times in the days before you go off, or your baby and babysitter may have a miserable time. Young babies usually prefer the milk to be lukewarm. The easiest way is to stand the bottle or cup in a large bowl of warm water for a few minutes. Some people use microwaves, but be wary of these because the milk may not heat evenly – the main worry is if there is a scalding hot spot. Shake the bottle then drip a bit onto the back of the hand to test.

Some manufacturers claim that their bottle teats are more breast-like than others, so that the baby can suckle in a similar way. Note that teats come in different flows – get a slow teat for a very young baby. Some women find that their babies actually start to prefer suckling from a bottle because the milk is dispensed more quickly. This "nipple confusion" is one reason why some people prefer to use cups than bottles.

It's not easy to tell how much expressed milk your baby is likely to want in the time that you will be away. You may find you need to express several times to satisfy one meal. Therefore, if you can, express several times over several days and store each session's milk in the freezer. Special pre-sterilised, disposable bags are available, into which a breastpump can directly dispense milk. They can then be frozen individually and brought out as needed, attaching to their special make of bottle.

Expressing is useful for helping to maintain full breastfeeding without having to resort to formula, and some women do it frequently with ease. But the reality is that many women find it hard and don't do it often.

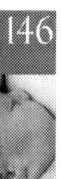

Some Stories About Expressing

Rosalyn: "I borrowed an electric breastpump, which could empty me in five or ten minutes compared with about 45 minutes of hand expressing. I started expressing at three weeks, because I had to go into work for a few hours every now and then whilst my boyfriend fed our daughter the expressed milk. It's a weird feeling to open the freezer and see sachets of your own milk. I expressed a lot and soon noticed a difference in volumes that would come out during a session, at first it might be just 1oz, later it was about 2oz or 4oz on a good day, and, on one occasion after I had been drinking Guinness, 7oz, which we were nervous to use! My boyfriend would thaw two, three or four packets at a time, depending on how hungry she seemed.

Sometimes I would express in the morning, when there was still milk to spare. Then because I would get very full whilst at work (up to five or six hours), I would express again on one side as soon as I got back home, while she had the other side as normal. It wasn't too bad a rhythm, several times a week, and we didn't use any formula at all for four months. Having said that, though, I wouldn't particularly recommend regular expressing to other women. The noise of the machine really got on my nerves and there were occasions when nothing would come out – stress – and I would become utterly frustrated and hurl the equipment across the room. On the last occasion that happened, at about six months, I quit. Also, my circumstances of working very flexibly part-time within a few months of birth are not the norm. I would say to any woman planning to return from maternity leave that expressing and work are not as compatible as breastpump manufacturers and breastfeeding books might have you believe, just another complicated facet of working motherhood…"

Vicky had bought a handpump, but found she was rarely away from her child to warrant using it. Annette, like many women, found expressing difficult: "I wanted to express so that my husband could do a late evening feed whilst I went to bed early. I tried various hand techniques and massaging motions that friends showed me, but hardly anything came out. I borrowed two pumps, which helped a bit, but only about a tablespoon's worth. After a couple of weeks of trying different things, and with me still feeling incredibly tired two months after the birth, we decided to do the late evening feed with a bottle of formula."

Introducing Formula Into the Equation

Supplementing with formula is rarely suggested by health advisers and may actually be discouraged – the amount of formula to breastmilk proportionately increases the risk of allergy and gastro-enteritis in the baby, whilst immune

Feeding Rhythms

SUCCESSFUL BREAST AND BOTTLE COMBINATIONS
If you want to continue with a combination of breast and bottles, you will need to stabilise the ratio:

- *Rather than offering bottles of formula after each breastfeed, substitute a whole feed. In this way, your baby is less likely to start fussing on the breast in anticipation of the bottle.*

- *Do the bottle feed(s) at roughly the same times each day, so your body can adjust more easily.*

- *Many women need a minimum of six breastfeeds in 24 hours to maintain a reasonable supply.*

- *Some women can stabilise supply with morning and evening breastfeeds. This might be your aim if returning to work.*

factors from breastmilk are proportionately decreased. However, many mothers start supplementing for a wide range of reasons relating to emotional and practical difficulties with breastfeeding and expressing. Some difficulties might be resolved if a woman has enough correct information and support with breastfeeding. Others might ultimately be unresolvable without scaling down breastfeeding, especially if a mother is mentally and physically distressed with the intensity of exclusive breastfeeding – a perhaps more common cause of unhappiness than is generally regarded. Unfortunately, because supplementing is usually a decision that the woman takes of her own volition without obvious support from health professionals (indeed, against the force of the pro-breastfeeding lobby), a certain amount of worry and guilt may ensue.

Sadly, many women find that when they start supplementing with bottles, a vicious circle of declining breastmilk supply soon begins, with the ratio quickly swinging to formula over breastmilk, even though they might have wanted to continue breastfeeding for longer. Dropping a breastfeed will make your breasts overfull, then they will scale down production. Some women's bodies can settle into a rhythm of one to three breastfeeds spaced through the day, but for others this is not enough stimulation to maintain milk production, and it "dries up". (Your baby might still like suckling for comfort, but the milk supply might be gradually dropping without you realising.) On the other hand, if you are aware of the potential problems, you might be able to avoid the circle that culminates in bottle-dependency. Many people do successfully combine breastfeeding and formula for many months and regard it as a good compromise (left panel).

One common reason given for starting supplementary bottles is a feeling that the milk supply is low towards the end of the day. Some parents decide to feed one bottle of formula in the evening in the hope that it will stave off some of the crying and help induce sleep. A common scenario is with a partner coming home from work and being pleased to have the opportunity to be involved with feeding once a day whilst the mother gets more rest.

Formula is heavier than breastmilk on the baby's stomach, thus it takes longer to digest (about 20% longer) and can induce a heavier sleep. This may seem an attractive proposition when you are craving more sleep, but it can sadly be a bit of a quick fix. Ultimately, a late-night feed of bulky formula interferes with sleep – rather than losing a dependency on night feeding, your baby's body learns to rely on it for volume and bulk. If you think of your adult feeding pattern, you would probably avoid a heavy meal before bedtime because indigestion might wake you up in the night. Therefore, supplementing in daytime is better unless your reason for supplementing is simply to get more sleep at night right now, which would also be understandable.

A Big Chapter About Feeding

Most parents who use formula get hooked on a certain brand, and the organic brands have become popular recently. Some come in liquid form, some as powder that has to be made up with cooled, boiled water. See Robin Barker's summary of Typical Patterns of Baby Behaviour (pp102–109) for the amount of formula that's needed at different ages.

Bottles have to be sterilised (see the methods mentioned in Expressing) to minimize the risk of gastro-enteritis, which is very debilitating for a young baby. However, once your baby has started to put all kinds of objects in her mouth, you might justifiably query why you have to keep sterilising the bottles. This is another subject on which there is no consensus. Most health advisers say to sterilise for 12 months; a few have said don't bother after six months. It actually depends on how much defence to gastro-intestinal bacteria your baby has developed, which of course is impossible to quantify unless you stop sterilising and find your baby gets a bug. It seems that most parents sterilise up to 12 months.

Some Stories about Feeding Rhythms
Rosalyn – a year of feeding

"Like a lot of first-time mothers, I was really surprised by the amount of time spent feeding. I think in the affluent West we forget how eating is for survival, but your newborn reminds you. I breastfed whenever she cried for the first six weeks or so, which was anything from 10 to 15 times at different intervals through the day and night. I didn't bother getting her weighed each week. She was so obviously thriving – fat belly and glowing skin. But I was so tired and longed for the relentless feeding to ease off. When I read somewhere that breastmilk takes about three hours to digest, I thought I would dare to try a routine. This involved waking her up if she napped more than two hours in a row during the daytime, and encouraging her to have a big feed before the next nap, rather than two or more little feeds.

Within a few days she had accepted the routine, every three hours or so. I would look at the clock and think "she's due for her mid-morning feed, or this is lunch, afternoon tea, the early evening feed, the night feeds". Sometimes there would be little snacks in between, but so long as she was having those main meals, I was happy and felt that the day was a bit more structured.

From about weeks six to ten, I remember feeding her at night as soon as she started making little noises, before she fully woke up, because it seemed that she would settle back to sleep quicker like that. However, after reading Richard Ferber's sleep book I realised that this was teaching her a bad habit, so after that I waited for her to cry at night. She soon started sleeping much longer at night without me giving her feeds that she didn't really need.

CUTTING DOWN ON BREASTFEEDING
When you want to scale down or stop breastfeeding, do so gradually – allow at least two weeks. Cut back on feeds one at a time. Hand express excess milk, so that your breasts do not become engorged. Mastitis is a possibility if you stop too suddenly.

Some women find that a tiny bit of foremilk can be expressed from their breasts long after they have stopped breastfeeding. Indeed, once lactation has been triggered in your body, it might never be totally suppressed. This is why some women have managed to reboost supply from virtually nothing – with very frequent suckling and expressing, the breasts get the signal to pump up the volume of milk again.

At about four months, she started sleeping more regularly for her daytime naps as well as at night, so I shuffled the feeding times a bit, into early morning, late morning, mid-afternoon, early evening and late evening feeds. I stopped offering her feeds if she woke up in the night around this time. We also started using formula alongside breastmilk, one bottle at lunchtime, with me breastfeeding morning and evening, a ratio that continued for another four months. At six months, her sleep pattern shifted again, with a really long sleep at night, and two quite long naps during the day. In between each nap would be the basic pattern of breakfast, lunch and supper, with milk and solids at each mealtime and maybe snacks at odd times. In fact this is exactly the same pattern we are in now, many months on. She usually drinks about the same amount of milk each day, but intake of other foods is incredibly variable: some days she'll eat everything, especially fruit and cakes; then for several days almost nothing."

Katie – changing patterns in the first four months

"Jack had problems latching on at the beginning. He would try but then pull away from me crying, which was no fun for either of us. I spent the first 10 days expressing for as much as an hour before every feed (sometimes he got angry waiting), then I would feed him the breastmilk in a bottle, which he would take about 15 minutes to get through. Can you imagine, I was doing this expressing about seven times a day? It was such a ridiculous situation. Fortunately, before I went totally mad, a friend recommended an NCT breastfeeding counsellor who actually came round to my house and helped him latch on.

He spent the next three days confused about the disappearance of the bottles and cried a lot, going on and off the breast, but I persisted and eventually he would settle to feed on the breast for about 20 minutes at a time. I would have relaxed, but colic hit a week later, and some evenings would be spent with him going on and off the breast and crying in between. My husband suggested that he could give Jack a bottle of expressed milk in the evening whilst I got some rest. So I would express about three times a day in between his feeds, in order to get enough milk for the evening. I was the Dairy Maid Supreme.

When Jack was about eight weeks old, I decided one day that I couldn't bear any more expressing and that he could have one bottle of formula in the evening. We did this for a month, and I felt better, actually enjoying breastfeeding without all the expressing. I was still tired from the night feeds, though. He dropped to one night feed at three months, but I then found that I had too much milk. The supply was very uneven between day and night. I thought it would be best if I dropped the mid-day breastfeed to match. So he's had two bottles of formula and two breastfeeds each day for the past month."

Nisha – three children, and three very different experiences

"My experiences might interest other mothers. I breastfed my first son for a year and had few problems after the nipple sensitivity wore off. He was naturally a settled baby and would feed well from both sides about seven or eight times a day. I knew that the positioning was important and that I shouldn't limit his feeds. He fed two or three times at night in the first three months – I would bring him into bed with me.

Back then, I will admit that I didn't have much sympathy for mothers who chose to bottle-feed. That was to change. My second son was born by caesarian three weeks early, weighing just 5lb 10oz, and he was very jaundiced for a few days. Not only was I suffering after the 36-hour labour and scar, but he wanted to feed every two hours, and I found this frequency very hard, especially with his older brother to care for at the same time. My health visitor said it was normal for a premature baby to want to feed more frequently because of the smaller stomach. But knowing this didn't help. I got very tearful and depressed, and those early months of having two children were extremely difficult. Fortunately, my own mother stepped in to do some feeding with formula or I would not have coped at all. I gave up breastfeeding at seven weeks, which I did feel was a shame for him, and he did get more upset stomachs and colds than his siblings. But better that than have his mummy carted off to an asylum.

With my third, a daughter, I had mentally prepared myself for a hard time, but she turned out to be an incredibly settled baby from the start, hardly any colic and sleeping through at about three months. Breastfeeding every three or four hours was not too difficult. That's not to say it was a breeze. At that time, I'd say at least three-quarters of the day was spent cooking, feeding and clearing up after the boys, and breastfeeding the baby. A mother's work is never done…

But then I had flu at three months, which somehow triggered mastitis in both breasts. That was the most awful experience, and it kept flaring up so I decided to cut right down on breastfeeding (which has to be done very gradually when you have had mastitis). I now understand and sympathise with women who give up breastfeeding early, and am totally in awe of mothers I know who have continued to breastfeed through mastitis and other problems."

Amy – breastfed both her children for over a year each

"I basically fed on demand. With my first child, I started to identify the "I'm hungry" cry in the first month. The number of feeds varied, from maybe 10 in 24 hours in the first four months, which gradually went down. By a year they were having three meals a day, plus maybe four or five breastfeeds. I never used formula, but after a year slowly weaned them onto cow's milk in a beaker."

A BIG CHAPTER ABOUT SLEEP

153

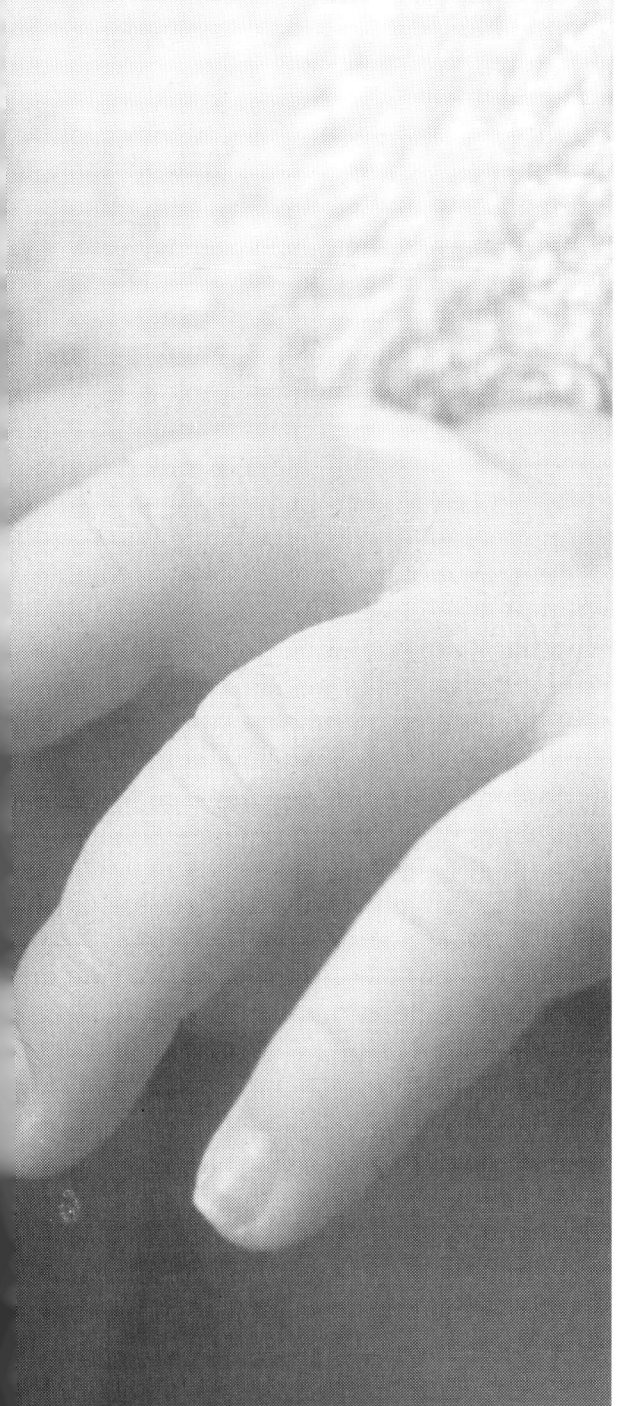

Contents

154 Sleeplessness and Tiredness

158 How We Sleep

162 Sleep Politics

168 Encouraging a Good Sleep Pattern

181 A Middle-Way Sleep Strategy

189 Stories about Sleep

195 Avoiding Cot Death

SLEEPLESSNESS AND TIREDNESS

The way in which sleep matures in the child and the impact of sleep deprivation on the parent are very significant in the early months. In this big chapter about sleep, we look at why mothers get so tired, how sleep works, the politics of where your baby sleeps, and a range of ideas on how to get more sleep.

A Mother's Tiredness

Ask a new mother about tiredness. We all expect broken nights with a baby, but until you experience it for yourself, it is impossible to guage how wearying life with a newborn will be. Looking at the workload – feeding, hygiene, etc – tells only a small part of the story. Other important factors are as follows:

You are weaker after birth Pregnancy was tiring in itself. Adrenaline and will power kept you going through labour and maybe the first few days, but even if your birth was straightforward it was still a tremendous physical feat that will have tired you out immensely. If you had a really hard, long labour, and particularly if you had a caesarian and major blood loss, then you may be extremely weak for some weeks to come. We enter motherhood in a state of tiredness but of course have no time to just rest and recuperate.

You are in at the deep end New experiences can be both exhilarating and tiring. If this is your first baby then not only have you just lived through the incredible experience of birth but also each day is bringing further new experiences, perhaps bizarre and scary. You are suddenly a parent and having to reorganize your life, finding new ways of doing things and continually learning as you go. Your mind will become really tired from all this sensory bombardment and from you trying to make sense of your new life.

You are constantly on call Having just made the astonishing transition from an existence within your womb to life outside, your baby is unsettled, feeding and sleeping in short bursts, swaying between hot and cold, and crying inexplicably. The unpredictability of this and the way you have to constantly watch over and listen out for the baby are wearying.

A Big Chapter About Sleep

Your night sleep is broken This is the most obvious reason why you are tired. To a certain extent your mind and body will adjust to interrupted sleep, but the general effect will be mildly disassociating – a feeling of never being entirely awake or on the ball. It exacerbates all the other reasons for tiredness.

You may have insomnia In late pregnancy many women find they awaken rather easily at night, maybe from discomfort. Insomnia after the birth is a sign of overstimulation and disruption to your internal rhythms, usually temporarily, but distressing in its own right. Resorting to sleeping pills at this time may complicate or prolong the problem, but your health visitor may have more advice.

Your hormones have just drastically changed Some will have plummeted shortly after the birth; others will be kicking in for breastfeeding and other things. Hormonal changes are often tiring (consider pre-menstrual syndrome!). There is also a theory that women's hormones put them on a constant state of alertness to any sign of distress in their children. So perhaps your baby only has to whimper for you to wake up, further disrupting your sleep. (Or the pressure in your breasts may wake you even if your baby sleeps on.)

Getting Through the Tiredness

In some ways, the suggestions that follow seem ridiculously obvious, but if you get into a state of exhaustion you may not be able to think straight or see the wood for the trees. It's even better to anticipate situations and avoid reaching a point of complete exhaustion. So here is a mixture of suggestions compiled from midwives, health visitors, yoga practitioners and mothers.

Get people to help you If the father of your baby is around for the majority of the day and night, then great (though don't be surprised if you still need extra help from other people). If he's working or going back to work within a few weeks of the birth, you may well need extra support during the day. Few new mothers get this extra support after their partners go back to work, but really it should be the norm.

On a very practical level, eating well after birth is important because of the demands on your body. But often the shopping for food, cooking it and clearing it up are just too complicated with a tiny child in tow. If you are one of the one-in-four women who had a caesarian, then you are temporarily disabled and not supposed to lift and carry for a few weeks. You shouldn't be expected to cope alone with a new baby in such circumstances, but some women find they have to. We need a sea-change in attitudes and more compassion for new mothers.

THE IMPACT OF SLEEP DEPRIVATION
Alice, one of the mothers interviewed by the editor, expresses the difficulties of the post-partum period:

"The only thing that matters in the early weeks is sleep. If you can get enough sleep, then you can cope with most other things. However, if you don't get enough sleep, then even the tiniest thing during the day is enough to push you over the edge."

Sleeplessness and Tiredness

There may be some parts of the babycare, such as soothing and bathing, that people close to you can help with while you rest. If you are fully breastfeeding, you could try expressing some milk to be given in a bottle while you get some unbroken sleep (see pp145–149). Make sure that the baby is out of earshot or you might wake up anyway and fret about not doing the feeding yourself.

In many cultures the extended family automatically helps to care for both mother and child. In our prevailing culture we may have to ask for help – and many mothers don't ask, and so become ever more tired and isolated. Even if you do have supportive people saying "can I do anything?", you may perceive it as a double-edged offer. You might crave advice and help but also want to do things, or try out things, in your own way – caring for the baby is wrapped up with bonding. One way round this is to make it as clear as possible what kind of help you would appreciate (though it may not be easy to predict).

If you don't feel you have enough supportive family and friends nearby, at least consider hiring some domestic help for a while. This should not be stigmatised as just the preserve of the rich. If shopping is difficult (in terms of negotiating transport, lifting and carrying etc), try places that do home delivery. Some of the major supermarkets have an Internet service and will deliver for around £5 per visit (see right panel). Avoiding a state of nervous exhaustion is worth any amount of extra expense in the short term…

Don't take on too much This is perhaps the most obvious piece of advice and yet the hardest to follow. What constitutes "too much" depends on your state of health and state of mind. You might know people who were out socialising with their babies or working within days of giving birth and want to emulate them, but you simply do not have the reserves of strength. In the earliest weeks you may find that you feel fairly ok one day but very tired the next. (Perhaps some of the new mothers you saw out and about overdid it and spent the next few days feeling shattered.) It's probably best not to make plans for anything much at this stage. Too many of us are competitive about motherhood – we feel that we have to prove to the world and ourselves that we can be supermums from the start.

A lot of second-time mothers have said that the early weeks with the second child were not as tiring as with the first, because they took life a lot easier…

Also bear in mind that you won't have such a sudden transition ever again in your life – you make the transition to motherhood only once. You may have to work out some new ways of doing things with subsequent children, but the learning curve is not nearly so steep and tiring. Just knowing that you are in the worst of it now can help you psychologically to get through the tiredness, which

---

THINGS THAT MIGHT HELP IF YOU HAVE INSOMNIA

• Every now and then get up, wander round the house, then go back to bed.

• Stop actually trying to sleep. Just lie with your eyes shut and your body in a state of deep relaxation.

• You may have developed a heightened sensitivity to noise – try wearing earplugs.

• If even small noises from the baby are keeping you awake, move the cot into another room.

• Herbal and homeopathic remedies for insomnia might help.

• Sleeping pills on prescription are never a good solution for long-term insomnia, but might help if you are desperate. Make sure your GP knows if you want to continue breastfeeding.

you might otherwise perceive as endless. And at whatever stage of motherhood you are, if tiredness is getting to you, just slow down as far as you can, and take each day as it comes...

Practice deep relaxation At various points in the day, when your baby is asleep, try lying down in a flat, balanced position, relax every muscle in your body and clear your mind for 10 to 20 minutes. This can be a surprisingly effective way to recharge yourself for a few hours at a time. Don't actually try to fall asleep in such a short amount of time otherwise you might start going into a deep sleep, which feels worse to come out of. Conversely you might feel frustrated at not being able to fall asleep.

If you have never tried this kind of relaxation before, perhaps concentrate on different sets of muscles at a time. Starting with the head, say, relax your scalp muscles, eye and jaw muscles, and move down to the neck, shoulders, back etc, down to your toes until every muscle in your body is relaxed. Listen intently to the sounds in the world around you: the breeze in the trees, gurgling in the pipes, faraway voices and so on. Or literally *concentrate* on relaxing your body. This will stop your mind from wandering onto thoughts about things that need to be done around the baby or things in your life that are beyond your control, which will stress your mind and make your body tense up again.

Sleep when your baby sleeps This is a common piece of advice and is meant to remind you that taking time to sleep is more important than catching up on things that have been pushed to one side while you have been nurturing the child. Then again, some people have pointed out that sleeping when the baby sleeps is quite hard to achieve. Not everyone can fall asleep at the drop of a hat, especially if the expectation is of being woken again quite soon. Also, your own physical and mental 24-hour cycle, used to sleeping a chunk at night, may not allow you to sleep during daytime (see circadian rhythms in the next section). So, unless you do have the ability to fall asleep very easily (in which case, go ahead), you may be better off practicing deep relaxation when your baby sleeps during the day. Keep sleep for the night, even if you anticipate it being broken. Maybe go to bed a lot earlier for now.

Encourage your baby into a rough 24-hour routine This is a controversial area, but if a lot of your tiredness boils down to the unpredictability and shortness of your baby's sleeps and seemingly endless feeds, then you might find that trying to coax them into a rough pattern works better than waiting for a pattern to emerge. For a lot more on this see pp87–90, 173–177.

HOME DELIVERY/ INTERNET SHOPPING
• www.sainsburys.co.uk
0845 301 2020

• www.tesco.com
0845 722 5533

• www.waitrose.com
0800 188 884

• www.johnlewis.com
08456 049 049

BABY PRODUCTS CATALOGUES
• www.bloomingmarvellous.co.uk
0870 751 8944

• www.jojomamanbebe.co.uk
0870 241 0560

Some of the parenting websites, such as listed on p82, offer online shopping.

How We Sleep

This section looks at the nature of sleep in babies and adults, and how sleep cycles and circadian rhythms mature. Understanding what scientific research has revealed about sleep can be helpful for parents during the early months with their newborns.

Types of Sleep

Sleep fluctuates through the night. There are different types of sleep stages and sleep cycles that all of us go through at night, whether we are aware of them or not when we wake the following day. Researchers have classified sleep into two basic types: REM and NON-REM. For the sake of clarity, they can be referred to here as dreaming sleep and deep sleep.

Deep sleep So-called non-REM sleep is associated with falling asleep and a deep, dreamless sleep. Scientists subdivide it into four levels of deepening sleep, each of which have quite distinct brainwave patterns. Once you reach the fourth level of deep sleep you will be at your most oblivious to the external world. It is thought that our bodies and minds rest and repair themselves the most during deep sleep.

Dreaming sleep It is called REM (rapid eye movement) sleep because your eyes will twitch a lot beneath your eyelids as you dream. Other parts of your body might also twitch. The brainwaves of dreaming sleep show it to be a state between deep sleep and wakefulness. Your metabolism also becomes quite active while you are dreaming.

Sleep Cycles in Adults

During an eight-hour night, an adult will typically go through the different types of sleep in several cycles. First come the four stages of dreamless sleep, taking you from wakefulness down to a very deep sleep. This might take an hour or an hour and a half. Then might follow a period of lighter, dreaming sleep. After this dreaming interlude you will probably go into a deeper sleep again, through another cycle of non-dreaming sleep stages. Your sleep then lightens again, and for most of the rest of the night you will fluctuate between dreaming and the lighter stages of non-dreaming sleep. Usually there is a short period of very deep sleep at about 5am, after which you will go back to dreaming and progressively lighter sleep until either you automatically wake up refreshed or an alarm clock lifts you out of the end stages of slumber.

About a quarter of adult sleep is spent dreaming, though you may not remember all your dreams the next morning. Moreover, as you go from one stage of sleep to another, especially from a very deep sleep to a light dreaming sleep, you will often partially wake up and turn over for a few minutes. Again, you won't necessarily remember these brief awakenings the next morning. But it is important to understand that sleep is never solid, not even in an adult, and certainly not in a newborn baby.

SLEEP CYCLES IN BABIES

Interestingly, sleep states approximating to REM and non-REM develop whilst babies are still in the womb. The dreaming sleep appears first and is the dominant one up to the eighth month of gestation. What we dream about in the womb is anyone's guess.

Unlike an adult, who will go through deepening stages of dreamless sleep first, the newborn baby enters dreaming sleep first and spends about half its sleep time in this state. The newborn's non-REM, or dreamless sleep, does not have the same stages as seen in an adult.

However, the brain continues to mature rapidly after birth. After just one month the dreamless sleep starts to take on the distinct subdivisions and cycles seen in an adult. By three months the baby is entering the deep, dreamless sleep first, followed by dreaming sleep, like an adult. Unlike an adult, though, the baby reaches the deepest state of sleep in about 10 minutes.

For daytime naps the three-month-old baby might complete just one cycle of sleep then wake up. At night-time, however, there will be several cycles, with brief awakenings in between each, much like an adult, but probably more active than an adult. Some babies learn how to settle themselves after these awakenings from a young age. They move around and maybe whimper a bit then go back to sleep on their own. Other babies don't know how to settle themselves back to sleep and may start crying. In the early weeks this will be a cue for a feed, but once your baby's digestive capacity has grown and is fulfilled by daytime feeds, the night feeds will not be necessary.

Once the dreamless sleep cycling has developed, some babies might partially wake from the deepest sleep in a state of confusion, screaming. This kind of sleep disturbance is more likely to occur in the early part of the night, one or two hours after your baby has gone to bed. The confusion might be worse if the surroundings are different to when the baby went to sleep (for instance, if he fell asleep in your arms before you transferred him to the cot). It's not a hunger cry, although you might mistake it for one.

By six months slumbering babies are showing all the same brainwave patterns and cycles as sleeping adults although the cycles vary in length from adult ones. This is not to say that all babies have automatically adopted a settled sleep pattern at this age, with a long, unbroken night sleep and predictable daytime naps. They may need your help with this in conjunction with their naturally maturing sleep processes. And, as most babycare writers like to point out, some children will continue to wake up regularly in the night for many years, despite the best efforts of parents to break the habit.

Circadian Rhythms

As well as understanding how sleep cycling works during the night, it's worth looking at the 24-hour sleep pattern to understand how sleep matures. Adults usually take their sleep in one go at roughly the same time each night. This 24-hour sleep-awake cycle is called a circadian rhythm. There are many other circadian rhythms – such as fluctuations in temperature, respiration, digestion activity, the workings of the immune system and especially the secretion of hormones – which ebb and flow in a 24-hour pattern.

Not all our biological cycles are over a 24-hour time period to match the turning of the Earth. A woman's ovulation-menstruation cycling, for instance, takes place over roughly 28 days. However, the 24-hour sleep-awake circadian rhythm is the foundation of the biological clock, helping to regulate all other bodily functions. Some biological activities are increased throughout the night, such as the secretion of melatonin; some peak at different stages of either deep or light sleep. For instance, cortisol in blood plasma (part of the immune system) typically peaks at about 6am, after the last cycle of deep sleep.

The biological clock in humans is helped partly by external cues such as lightness and darkness. Within the retina of the human eye are light receptors that send messages to parts of the brain's hypothalamus and pineal gland, which trigger the release of various chemicals that govern the biological rhythms. Studies have shown that these chemicals still get released in cyclical patterns if some of the cues are absent, but the overall time lengthens slightly. For example, in a famous test by sleep researchers in the 1960s, subjects living in a bunker for a few weeks without natural light or a clock actually slept and woke in a 25-hour rhythm, and their other biological rhythms were lengthened.

When circadian rhythms get disrupted in adults – such as when you travel east or west to a different time zone, or if you do shift work – the overall effect

A Big Chapter About Sleep

is of feeling either tired or wakeful at an inappropriate time of the day. The effects of jet lag can last for a fortnight until your body fully adjusts its circadian rhythms to suit the new sleep-wake times. All bodily functions will be under duress as they attempt to adapt to the new rhythm. Your immune system and digestion will not work so well, and your mental agility will be lowered.

How Circadian Rhythms Develop

Newborn babies do not have circadian rhythms. If they have any *in utero*, linked to the maternal rhythms, they appear to lose them when they leave the sanctuary of the womb. At birth and for the first few weeks their sleep-awake times, digestion and other biological secretions are mostly random. By about six weeks of age, however, some of the biological rhythms are taking on a 24-hour pattern. By about 16 weeks the circadian rhythms are highly developed in many babies. The underlying 24-hour pattern is then set for life, though the details will change and adapt to different circumstances throughout life.

It is not known exactly how big a part social cues (such as parents instigating a 24-hour routine) and environmental cues (such as daylight, air temperature changes, noise levels) play in the development of circadian rhythms in the first 16 weeks of life. However, they will all help to reset the biological clock, synchronizing it with Earth's spin rather than free-running to more than 24 hours. Adults use cues such as alarm clocks and creating a certain set of conditions (comfy bed, darkness etc) to refine their sleep-wake cycle. Babies need adults to help refine the cycles. However, this leads into the arena of sleep politics – where babies should sleep and whether or not it is acceptable to instigate a routine.

Because newborn babies do not have underlying circadian rhythms, the randomness of their sleep-wake and other cycles does them no harm. This is why we are told in some babycare books that very young babies get all the sleep they need, even if the parents think the child is surely not getting enough. In fact, it is the parents themselves who are suffering. Constantly broken nights mean that night-time hormonal secretions are confused, digestion altered, the immune system weakened – an immense stress on the body and mind of an adult. Likewise, once babies have developed circadian rhythms, disruption to those rhythms can cause similar stress. Older babies and children can suffer from not having enough sleep – irritation and hyperactivity are well-known symptoms. Babies soon develop the capability of keeping themselves awake from excitement or if sleeping conditions don't seem right. Eventually you will probably have to take some kind of initiative to coax your baby into and maintain the circadian rhythms. Ways to do this are covered later in this chapter.

GOOD BOOK ON SLEEP
The best-known book on babies' sleep patterns is Solve Your Child's Sleep Problems, by Dr Richard Ferber. For more about this, see p82.

SLEEP POLITICS

*S*leep has become an arena for opposing views. Where your baby sleeps and how much you can, should or shouldn't try to steer your baby into a sleep routine are sources of contention. Unfortunately, many popular babycare books today either give just one line of advice or leave out such sleep topics. Here is a summary of the main issues.

BRINGING THE BABY INTO YOUR OWN BED

You might assume that your own bed would be a hazardous place for the newborn. After all, the official advice for avoiding cot death – placing babies on their backs at the bottom of the cot, keeping the room temperature at about 18 degrees etc (see p196) – gives an impression that babies need a very regulated environment in which to sleep. In fact, there is no official directive from the health authorities saying that you mustn't let your baby sleep with you in your own bed.

On the other hand, there may not be an official "no" to bed-sharing, but there are some official words of caution. Because smoking is one of the biggest risk factors with SIDS, if you or your partner are smokers then you are warned against bringing the baby in with you at night. This is not just if you smoke in bed – any residue of smoke on your body from elsewhere will be in that much closer proximity to your sleeping baby. Another risk factor is if you use a duvet – this would be too hot for the baby. And if either you or your partner are heavy sleepers or have been drinking, then don't sleep with the baby. The danger with this last one is not from SIDS, but from crushing.

Besides these factors, research so far has not definitively shown bed-sharing to carry a greater risk of SIDS (sudden infant death syndrome).

But the advice and politics don't end there. Some childcare gurus, particularly attachment theorists in America (e.g. William Sears, see p83) say that babies and children should sleep in bed with you, not in a cot, for the sake of bonding. This advice has been highly influential in some circles. These gurus have studied family life in cultures where family bed-sharing is the norm. The idea is put forwards that babies are more likely to grow up secure and happy if they sleep with their parents rather than separated in a cot. An extreme child-centred approach, it proposes that you wait for your child to decide for himself when he wants to sleep separately from you.

Some of the proponents of bed-sharing refer to research that suggests babies are actually less likely to die of SIDS if they sleep with their parents. Reasons that have been proposed for this include the parents being more receptive to any difficulties the baby might have with breathing or overheating, or that the rhythm of adult breathing is somehow transferred to the baby. But researchers are not in agreement about the interpretation of data from such studies. Indeed, when the editor contacted the Foundation for the Study of Infant Deaths to ask for their view about these theories, they stated that any such studies have not yet been supported by their own body of research. The jury is still out for the time being.

Where does this leave the ordinary parent who doesn't have preconceived ideas about where the baby should sleep? Parents often find that the baby falls asleep happily in their arms but cries when put in the cot or moses basket. As some breastfeeding experts point out, having the baby in bed with you means that night-feeding might be much easier. You can breastfeed while lying down, half-asleep, and both you and your baby might be able to fall asleep again after the feed, without having the disturbance of being transferred back to the cot.

But the bed-sharing advice throws up more issues and practicalities to consider. Family co-sleeping in other cultures (Thailand is one example) can involve parents and offspring sleeping together right up until the time that the children marry and move away. Our culture places a lot of emphasis on independence so few of us would seriously consider this to be an ideal option. Another practicality is that within a few months, babies start rolling around – you will need a big bed. If you are truly emulating other cultures then you will have to take the legs off your bed in case the baby rolls off.

Then there is an opposite line of advice from some babycare experts that it is best to avoid bringing the baby into your own bed. Instead, encourage your baby to get used to the cot from the start. Be consistent: don't have the child in bed with you one night and in the cot the next. Don't bring the baby into your bed midway through the night in order to feed. Avoiding these things will help speed up the process of consistent sleep conditioning so that your baby will eventually settle easier at night.

Family-bed proponents say that discouraging your baby from sleeping with you is unnatural, harsh and unloving. But the cot proponents say that some separation is actually better for the baby's emotional development – he learns from the start that he can be safe and secure sleeping away from you.

Sleep Politics

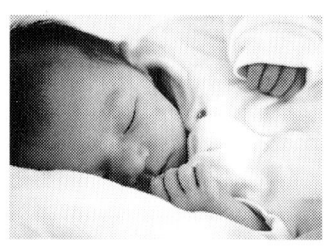

Sleeping peacefully on a nest of pillows, newborn Annie Foo is oblivious to the politics of co-sleeping versus cots.

Reading this, you might wonder: is it such an either/or issue? Is it not possible to switch your baby between cot and your own bed as you see fit? A lot of mothers try out both in the early weeks. Maybe you put the baby in the cot at the beginning of the night, then bring her into bed for a feed in the early hours and fall asleep together. It can be bliss at first, slumbering embraced in the comfort of each other's bodies. On the other hand, some parents sleep worse with the baby in bed with them – from worry about crushing and from being disturbed by the noisy, erratic breathing and jerky movements.

Within weeks, as sleep conditioning (see p176) starts taking hold in your baby's mind, you may find that you have to decide one way or another – whether you would prefer your baby to get used to her own cot now, or whether some or much of her sleep is going to be with you for many months or quite possibly years to come.

Cot, Cotbed, Crib or Basket?

Whether you should use a rocking crib, moses basket or suitable box for the first few weeks before transferring to a cot is an issue relating to the bonding theories as well as affordability. From both practical and financial points of view, a cot will be a suitable bed for your baby from birth up to the age of about two when she learns how to climb out. Cots sold in Britain meet certain safety standards, and most have mattresses that can be adjusted in height from high to low as the baby gains mobility. Cotbeds do not have adjustable heights but are larger and sturdier and can later be converted to a small bed lasting up to the age of about seven.

Cribs, baskets and other small cradle-like beds are popular items, but they don't last long. Babies quickly gain strength to roll and flail around and may outgrow them long before actually filling their size. However, baby-centred manuals encourage you to use a crib or basket first. The underlying assumption behind this advice seems to be that you will want your newborn right next to you at night without literally being in your arms all night – a sort of compromise between your own bed and a cot. There is also some kind of worry that a cot, with its bars and big, open space around the tiny baby, is too cell-like. The smaller basket or crib looks cosier, more reassuring.

From the parents' point of view, perhaps not so concerned with the theories about where babies feel most secure, the baby looks incredibly sweet in a tiny bed (though who these days seriously likes all those frills and drapes that come with them?). Rocking cribs might help with soothing, and a basket is easily transported around the house if you want to keep a constant close eye.

However, some people say that there is no psychological benefit in using a basket or crib rather than a cot to begin with. In fact, rather than feeling safer in

A Big Chapter About Sleep

a more enclosed space, the baby can only look upwards at the ceiling, unable to see you or anything much else and so may feel abandoned! Furthermore, your baby may become a little unsettled a few months down the line when you have to make the transition from cradle to cot. A further point is that there is nothing to stop you putting a cot right next to your bed if you want to partially emulate the family bed conditions. Indeed, some cots have a removable side designed for precisely this purpose.

Sleeping in Separate Rooms

Another level of sleep politics is whether the cot or cradle should be in the same room as you. Close proximity means that you will wake up easily when your baby starts whimpering. You might be able to breastfeed and resettle her with the mimimum of disturbance. You are not going to the extreme of sleeping with her in your arms, but you assume that she will know that you are right there nearby. Many of us have fears that our baby might die of cot death alone in another room (see p197). The drawback of sleeping in the same room, however, is that your baby's sometimes noisy breathing and snorts and partial awakenings might disturb you if you are a light sleeper. You may find yourself to be just as paranoid about cot death when you realise how irregular her breathing is. You may also find yourself having to resort to tiptoeing around. You and/or your partner may start to resent the baby's constant presence at night.

If your baby is in another room the occasional whimpers are less likely to wake you up and so she may resettle herself without needing to be fed or rocked. Her ability to resettle herself without your help becomes crucial as the months go by (see p178). Most mothers wake up easily when the whimpers become cries. You could use a monitor to be sure of waking, though whimpers and gurgles can sound harsh and ominous through a monitor, so you may find yourself waking up as much as if the baby was right next to you.

Parents tend to try out different things in relation to sleep, and ultimately the place(s) where you let your baby sleep should be the outcome of whatever you and your family are happiest with.

Links Between Breastfeeding Politics and Sleep Politics

Sleeping and feeding are closely linked in newborn babies, and sleep politics overlap with breastfeeding politics. It's worth knowing that many pro-breastfeeding activists and writers are proponents of the family-bed ideal, though the majority of parents in our country do not subscribe to this. Modern babycare manuals usually suggest three ways to help breastfeeding mothers deal with night feeds: to feed in bed so that you can remain half-asleep; to sleep when the baby does during the day, and perhaps to express some breastmilk for someone else to feed the baby while you sleep. Measures like these appear to help some mothers immensely, but not all. Some women interviewed for this book found that the disturbance of night feeds was not greatly lessened if done in bed rather than in a chair; sleeping in daytime was rarely easy (see p157); and expressing was hard work in itself.

The frequency of feeds and other variable factors will play a part in the mother's experience. A woman whose baby is waking to feed three or four times a night is bound to be suffering more from sleep deprivation than the mother of a baby who wakes up just once. A mother who is still suffering the effects of a hard labour may find the night feeds that much harder to cope with. Some women decide to mix breastfeeding and formula feeding because they are literally exhausted from breastfeeding. They might want to go somewhere else (perhaps just to bed for a longer stretch of unbroken sleep) while someone else feeds the baby. However, this strategy is rarely proposed in breastfeeding literature because it compromises the ideal of breastfeeding and can set in motion the circle of declining milk supply (see p148). Introducing formula is often discussed in terms of "choice" – the choice of the woman who doesn't want to breastfeed, or who wants to go out for the evening, or off to work. In some of the more extremist pro-breastfeeding writings is the idea that choosing to use formula compromises an ideal of maternal self-sacrifice. For some mothers, though, getting other people to help with feeding can be the difference between coping with tiredness or becoming exhausted and depressed.

BABY-LED VERSUS ADULT-LED SLEEP PATTERNS

The issue of sleep is bound up with the controversial issue of routines (see pp85–90). Should you always let your baby sleep whenever he likes and hope for a sleep pattern to develop of its own accord, as the baby-centred writings suggest? Some people fervently believe that you must follow the baby's lead because all babies are different and it would be cruel to impose a routine on a baby who doesn't want to fit into one. But can you steer the way with sleep from an early age as the routine-lovers propose? Many parents believe that the onus should be on the adult to lead the way or else bad sleep habits may build up. Scientific research into circadian rhythms supports the view that adult help is needed to keep a child's sleep-wake cycles on course each day. Probably most parents start out following the baby's lead, then find ways to coax the baby's sleep habits into a routine that suits the household.

A Big Chapter About Sleep

Parents' Views on Sleep Politics

The editor asked some parents for their views on where babies should sleep. Jacqui's awareness of sleep politics had begun on the maternity ward, the day after birth. "One of the midwives saw me napping with the baby on top of me and said I was spoiling her. I was flabbergasted by this attitude – how on earth can dozing together possibly be spoiling a baby? I didn't know about sleep politics at that stage, not until a couple of months went by and I discovered that some parents sleep with their children in bed with them for many years. That wouldn't be our choice. I'm glad she can't get out of her cot, though I guess when she's older she'll be running into our room in the middle of the night. But I think the midwife's attitude was too harsh. When you have just had a new baby you feel everyone is watching you and being judgemental, and this proves that they are. It's just too much pressure."

Maria and Ewan had bought a cot, but when interviewed at two months were finding it difficult to settle baby Callum in it and grappling with the issue. "He really hates being laid down, though we have tried warming up the sheets with a hairdryer and laying him in it very gradually. That's how it has been for the past few weeks. We can now see why people end up sleeping with their babies, and we sometimes do after a 4–5am feed."

Amy said that she had been heavily influenced by Deborah Jackson's *Three in a Bed* (see p91) and had strong views on the subject. "I would recommend co-sleeping to any parent. In fact, bed-sharing is natural, while cots are unnatural. When he sleeps with you, the baby can breastfeed whenever he wants in the night, and there is generally less disturbance." But Teresa was in disagreement on this point. "I was totally put off the family-bed idea because a friend and his wife had split up over this issue: she always wanted the baby in bed with them, but he found that unbearable, and I don't blame him. You need to spend time alone as a couple as well as in a threesome with the baby."

In the meantime, Siobhan expresses a seemingly common misgiving about the practicalities of bed-sharing: "I have absolutely no idea how some parents manage to sleep with their children in bed with them all night. We tried it in the first fortnight, but there is no way of sleeping with little fists and feet pummelling you every 20 minutes, pushing you to the edge of the bed. Also, if I did manage to fall asleep I would then wake up in a panic, thinking I had smothered her. I decided that she was going to have to get used to her cot, even if this meant having to get out of bed to breastfeed. There was often a bit of crying at bedtime to begin with, but she hasn't made a fuss for ages now. If you have a second bedroom, I would recommend using the cot in the nursery from birth. It's ridiculous to say that sleeping separately is cruel."

Encouraging a Good Sleep Pattern

There may be polarised views about baby-led versus adult-led sleep patterns, but you need not look at it as an either/or issue. Most babies eventually seem to settle into a pattern that is partly baby-led and partly parent-led. It's just a matter of degrees. This section looks at various ways in which you might encourage your baby to settle into a good sleep pattern as soon as possible.

BANDS OF NORMAL TOTAL SLEEP
Estimates vary in different sources. There seems to be a wide band of normality at newborn stage, which narrows with age.

- Newborn:
9 to 18 hours in maybe six to eight bursts. About 16 hours typical.
- One month:
12 to 18 hours, about 16 hours typical.
- Three months:
12 to 18 hours, about 15 hours typical.
- Six months:
12 to 17 hours, about 14 hours typical.
- Eighteen months:
12 to 16 hours, about 13.5 typical.
- Two years:
About 13 hours.
- Three years:
About 12 hours.
- Five years:
About 11 hours.
- Ten years:
About 10 hours.

How Much Sleep Do Babies Need?

If you add up all the hours of sleep that your baby has over each 24-hour period, you should find that the total is roughly the same each day and falls into the band of normality (see panel). Newborn babies do not have circadian rhythms (pp160–161), so the sleep they take in 24 hours is the amount that they need. This is why a newborn baby taking less than average sleep is not a problem for the baby. However, it may be a problem for an exhausted parent who may have to deal with a greater proportion of crying than average.

As the baby's sleep cycling matures and his ability to keep himself awake from excitement increases, he might start to suffer from too little sleep. There's no definitive age given by the popular manuals as to when a child might stop automatically taking the amount of sleep needed and when this might affect mental performance and behaviour. But it's widely acknowledged that within a few months of birth, most babies start having difficulty shutting out the world in order to fall asleep. Some parents claim this to be the case from birth.

Working out the average total hours that your newborn is taking – and so needs – does not, of course, take into account the way in which the sleep occurs in every 24 hours. A tiny minority of babies appear to be relatively settled in their sleeps at birth. But kipping in bursts of anything from 10 mintues up to three or four hours at a time in a wildly unpredictable manner is more typical newborn behaviour. There's no distinction between night and day sleeps, no pattern from one day to the next. With varying amounts of encouragement on your part, though, your baby can gradually settle into a sleep pattern whereby the majority of the sleep – however many hours it is in total – takes place at night, and the daytime sleeps are shortened to naps.

A Big Chapter About Sleep

What is a Settled Sleep Pattern?

An older, "settled" baby will have a predictable pattern of sleeps in a 24-hour period. "Settled" is in quotes because parents have different ideas as to what they consider settled, and the length and timing of sleeps vary from baby to baby even when they have adopted a pattern. For example, you might consider your baby settled as soon as you can see a pattern of sleeps, even if the pattern includes regular night feeds. Or you might consider your baby settled when his longest sleep corresponds with your own seven or eight hours. Or you might consider him settled only when the whole night from early evening to early morning is unbroken and daytime naps are predictable. A settled sleep pattern might also be dependent on a settled feeding pattern, with the majority or all feeds taking place in daytime.

For the purposes of this book and the sake of averages, "settled" means a long sleep at night – up to 12 hours without feeding or crying – and two or three daytime naps that might range from 20 minutes to three hours each in a fairly predictable pattern. This kind of pattern wouldn't be timed to the minute and would not preclude a disturbed night here and there, or stretch of days when naps or bedtimes go awry. Otherwise, it would be reasonably predictable, a good pattern for child and parents.

The occasional baby seems to adopt a pattern of taking all sleep during the night and none in the day, but this would be an unrealistic expectation of the vast majority of babies. Moreover, childcare and sleep experts are adamant that healthy children need daytime naps as well as a long night sleep up to the age of at least two, if not three or four.

Interestingly, sleep patterns in settled babies seem to be culturally driven in part. A 10- to 12-hour sleep at night, with one to three naps during the day is common for babies in Britain, North America and some parts of Europe. In some other countries such as Spain and in many Asian cultures a more typical pattern is for a shorter night sleep, but longer naps in the day and early evening, particularly with an afternoon "siesta". In such cultures, children might go to bed at about the same time as their parents, and their sleep patterns are almost certainly linked to a different pace of life generally.

When Do Babies Settle into a Pattern?

The question of "when" comes with caveats. Some people talk of definitive stages at which babies either can or should or are likely to settle. But there are many variable factors. The lengths to which you encourage a sleep pattern in the earliest months of your baby's life and your baby's receptiveness to this encouragement is a big factor. The rate at which the baby's brain and stomach

Encouraging a Good Sleep Pattern

capacity are maturing and the needs of other family members are amongst others. But even with all these variables, it's good to have an idea of what age babies typically settle into a sleep pattern. At the earliest end of the spectrum, you hear stories of some babies settling at four to six weeks. These babies will either be naturally heading into a pattern of sleep that suits their parents or they will be responding quickly to parental encouragements to settle.

Most childcare gurus are more conservative and say that three to four months is a more likely age at which a baby will (or can) settle into a sleep pattern that does not involve night feeds. Again, babies that settle around the age of three to four months may be a combination of those who are naturally disposed to settling and those who have been encouraged to adopt a pattern by their parents.

Six months is often cited as an age that the majority of babies are in a regular sleep pattern. The experts assure us that by six months babies should not need to feed at night although it is possible that some will still wake up in the night to feed out of habit – it has become their only way of getting back to sleep again (see the sections following sleep conditioning on pp176–180). Six months can thus be regarded as a bit of a benchmark. If your baby is still waking up regularly at night and taking ages to settle at this age (and a substantial number do), then you possibly have a long-term problem. A pattern may have developed, but it has "settled" as a pattern of waking at night. Either you haven't been giving enough encouragements to your baby to sleep through the night and with regular daytime naps, or you have given plenty of encouragements but your baby is stubbornly not taking to it.

Of course, the problem is only a problem if you perceive it as such – some parents regard disturbed sleep as inevitable whatever the age of the child and are not too worried by regular night awakenings or varying sleep times for the next few years. Or some perceive it as an ongoing inconvenience that, to some extent, they have got used to. If you do regard it as a problem, though, then sleep training might help, the sooner the better. If you have an older child who is hyperactive, often irritable or underperforming in mental, physical and social development, then it's also worth looking at whether lack of sleep or disturbed sleep is a factor.

As the weeks go by following birth, you may find that there are sudden breakthroughs with the development of a pattern of sleep. Perhaps, at a couple of months old, the baby suddenly starts sleeping a longer stretch at night, perhaps for seven or eight hours. A few weeks after this initial breakthrough there may be another in which, say, the daytime sleeps become more regular. Another month down the line there may be another development in which the

SETTLED BY EIGHT MONTHS?
The editor's local sleep clinic run by health visitors suggests that six to eight months is the benchmark for sleep maturation, both at night and during the day. The sleep training methods covered in this book are recommended by many health visitors and sleep experts. Consult your own health visitors if you continue to have sleep problems after eight months. They might be able to come up with a sleep training programme geared to your individual circumstances.

night sleep becomes longer still – the feed in the early hours gets dropped of its own accord, and the baby starts sleeping for ten to twelve hours at night.

Once a pattern of a long night sleep and two or three daytime naps has been established (hopefully by six months, if not sooner), it is likely to remain in place for many months. When the baby becomes a toddler the second or third daytime nap is usually the first to be dropped. By the age of three or four, most children will have dropped all daytime naps. By contrast, the 10- to 12-hour night sleep often seems to remain in place for many years. From maybe the age of eight or nine, bedtime gets put back progressively into the teenage years until the adult norm of eight hours sleep at night. (Not everyone follows this pattern, of course, it is just the typical average in our culture.)

As noted already, whether the sleep pattern is as quick to develop or eventually as "settled" as you might hope for might depend in part on how much encouragement you give in the crucial weeks when a pattern is developing. The sections that follow this cover a variety of ways in which parents nowadays encourage their babies to adopt a good sleep pattern.

Helping Your Baby to Distinguish Between Night and Day

The first positive thing you can do is encourage your baby to sleep a greater ratio of hours at night while the daytime sleeps are shortened to naps. If you are lucky then within a few weeks your baby will start sleeping for longer stretches at night than in the day with these most basic of encouragements. You will probably still have to do night feeds, but hopefully the baby will readily fall asleep again after the nocturnal snacks. Think in terms of giving your baby daily hints that daytime is for serious eating, activity and napping; night-time is for serious sleeping and sleepy snacking if need be. The methods are a mixture of tips from babycare manuals, health visitors, sleep experts and, not least, parents.

Keep night-time low-key Keep the light dim and diffuse when feeding your baby, only speak very quietly and generally don't actively try to engage with your baby. Avoid getting toys out or distracting the child with stimuli such as television – the idea is to make night seem less exciting in the way that you would during the day. In the earliest weeks it may be easiest to try quietly feeding-to-sleep or cuddling-rocking when the baby wakes up in the night, but at some stage in the not-too-distant future you are well advised to start encouraging your baby to fall asleep without these aids all the time.

You can instigate this kind of distinction between night and day as soon as you like after birth. But it's only a basic encouragement on your part, so don't

Encouraging a Good Sleep Pattern

expect your baby to make an immediate, miraculous differentiation between night and day just because it's darker, quieter and more boring for a long stretch of hours.

Blackout the room This is one of the more controversial tips. Some parents find that blacking out the baby's room helps the child to settle to sleep more easily than in a dimly lit room. The idea here is that even low lights or chinks of light might distract the child from sleep, and that complete darkness is more comfortably womblike. Guru Gina Ford (see p82) recommends blackouts. However, plenty of parents – probably the majority – don't like the idea of blackouts and don't find them necessary either. If you were afraid of the dark in your own childhood then you are unlikely to want to make your baby's room pitch black. There is also the possibility that if blackouts do work, then the baby may come to depend on absolute darkness in order to sleep – a nuisance when you are staying somewhere else. On the other hand, you could use blackouts to begin with, then gradually stop using them once a settled sleep pattern has emerged.

Put the baby to bed in the same place each night During the day you might want to let the baby sleep in all kinds of locations – in a baby chair, on a nest of cushions, in a pram, in a sling, in the car, in your arms, on top of you in your own bed etc. To help distinguish night from day, however, consider using just one location for the whole night – a crib, moses basket or cot in a particular room. (If you want to encourage regular daytime naps, too, consider using just one location for all sleeps.)

Feed more often during the day In order to minimize your baby's need for night feeds, in daytime try feeding your baby every two to three hours and as fully as possible each time – load up that little stomach to capacity. This might mean slightly bending, or broadening, the rule to "feed on demand", because you might sometimes want to offer a feed before the baby starts "demanding". You might even want to wake up the baby in order to feed every three hours minimum.

Feeding more during the day is not suddenly going to cancel out the need for night feeds, but it is another positive thing you can do to encourage things in the right direction.

Develop a bedtime ritual This is a delightful part of childhood in our culture and some other parts of the world. Work out some kind of ritual to do each evening that signals winding-down and bedtime to your baby. Popular things include a bath (even if one isn't needed), then a song or quiet game or story for an older baby, then dimming of the lights. Avoid boisterous games or any new stimuli. Doing the same calming activities at about the same time each evening are the key. Elements of the ritual can change over time, as can the person doing the ritual. If you want, you can incorporate a feed-to-sleep at the end of the ritual for a very young baby, but bear in mind that by the time babies are a few months old it is best if they can learn to settle themselves without having to be fed or rocked to sleep all the time.

Again, you can instigate a bedtime ritual as soon as you want after the birth. As with the other suggestions, it may not have much effect at first – in fact, you may feel rather ridiculous going through a seemingly pointless ritual only to have huge difficulty settling the baby afterwards. Nor will it automatically stop your baby from waking up later on. However, along with keeping night-time low-key, you are further reinforcing the idea that night is different from day. Furthermore, the bedtime ritual becomes something that both you and your child can hopefully really enjoy for years to come – a beautifully close and loving time of day, helping both of you to wind down and relax.

Swaddle or otherwise don't be obsessed with coverings Swaddling can be an excellent alternative to a sheet and blankets for very young babies, giving warmth, tactile comfort and a much greater sense of security (see p101). It can be one of the best ways of helping to induce sleep and minimizing the risk of the "startle" reflex waking up your baby.

If you don't like the idea of swaddling, bear in mind that the pictures in babycare manuals of babies sweetly tucked beneath a sheet and two blankets at the bottom of their cot are a laughably long way from the reality as most parents find it. Many newborn babies are quite capable of kicking off their covers within seconds, and this ability will only increase as the baby gains in strength. Parents can find themselves endlessly retucking blankets. Forget it. Check the temperature chart on p196 (note that overheating, rather than coolness, is regarded the risk factor with cot death – unless your house is very cold, then the baby will not suffer through having kicked off the covers). Can you put an extra layer of clothing on the baby rather than bothering with blankets at all? Some parents buy the special "sleeping bags" for babies rather than go through the nightly rigmarole of blanket adjusting.

Encouraging Regular Sleep Times

Like all the other mammals on the planet, we learn to live in 24-hour cycles with the turning of the Earth (see circadian rhythms on pp160–161). But whereas the changing pattern of darkness and light in every 24 hours, fluctuating

Encouraging a Good Sleep Pattern

temperatures and the turning of the seasons are the cues to other animals to sleep and wake, hunt and hibernate, mate and migrate, humans have developed the sophisticated cue of the 24-hour clock.

If you want to steer your baby a bit more towards a predictable pattern of sleeps, try encouraging sleep at certain times. This goes more into the realm of parent-led initiatives and routines than just creating different night and day conditions for your baby. So these tips, which come more from problem-solving sleep experts than the baby-centred gurus, are more controversial. Your baby might happily start sleeping and waking at certain times, in which case, great, but what if he or she doesn't? You may find that you have to try different solutions for different sets of circumstances. Sometimes you might want to persist in trying to settle the baby at a certain time, sometimes you might want to give up on that particular nap but try again later in the day and adjust other sleep times to fit. Sometimes you might be prepared to listen to some crying in the hope that your baby will shortly cry herself to sleep. Eventually, a 24-hour pattern emerges that is partly instigated by you, partly led by the baby.

You may have to apply different solutions for different circumstances even when a basic pattern has emerged. Your baby starts depending on cues. Some days your baby will be more sleepy and want to go to bed earlier. Some days you might want to bend the routine yourself and keep the baby up for longer than usual. And so on. But you still have your regular sleep times, the foundation of which you should be able to return to without much difficulty.

Set a bedtime in the early evening Given that newborn babies sleep for short bursts around the clock, you may feel it is ludicrous to set a particular time for bed in the evening for a very young baby. However, putting your baby to bed at the same time each night after a bedtime ritual strongly reinforces all the other signals to your baby that night-time is different from daytime.

As mentioned earlier, once settled, babies may remain in the same sleep pattern for many months, if not years. A baby sleeping for 10 to 12 hours at night is quite common in our culture. Therefore, set a bedtime in the evening at, say, 7.30 pm. At first this will make laughably little or no difference to the number of times your baby wakes up in the night or what time you find yourself getting up the next morning. But it helps your baby get used to a 12-hour night from the start and may speed up the process of settling into a sleep pattern.

If an early evening bedtime for your baby seems too ridiculous, you can try setting a late evening bedtime – the same time that you regularly go to bed perhaps. Then when your baby does start to sleep longer at night, you can gradually bring the bedtime forwards by several hours. However, this is a bit more confusing for a baby. Also, some parents have reported that the baby wakes up about the same number of times in the night regardless of whether they went to bed early or late.

Conversely, if you set an early evening bedtime in the early weeks, you may find that the baby starts taking the longest sleep in the evening and still wakes up in the middle of the night to feed. You can stick with this until the baby is sleeping the whole way through the night – at least you get the evening to yourself undisturbed. Or you can try waking up the baby for a sleepy feed just before you go to bed – the baby might then sleep longer in the early hours.

Some parents – a minority in our country – never set a particular bedtime, either in waiting for the baby to find his own night-time sleep pattern or because they do not perceive broken sleep to be a problem or because they don't mind if there is no set bedtime throughout childhood. That's fine, too. This part of the book will be of no interest if that is your way of thinking.

Encourage regular daytime naps As well as encouraging your baby to sleep 10 to 12 hours at night you can look at the timing and duration of daytime naps, too. This takes you another step into the realm of routines. A lot of parents set a fairly definite bedtime at night, then are happier to follow their baby's lead on daytime sleeps. If your baby's total sleep over 24 hours is about 16 hours, then you can eventually expect to see two or three daytime naps of one or two hours each in addition to 10 to 12 hours at night. If your baby's total sleep is a lot less than 16 hours then the daytime naps may be fewer and shorter and the night sleep may never reach 12 hours, but you should still be able to find a pattern of a long night sleep and one or two daytime naps.

Even if your baby's total sleep is 16 hours, try waking the baby up if a daytime nap goes beyond two-and-a-half or three hours. This is because at a few weeks of age many babies begin to sleep for a longer stretch just once in 24 hours – you want this longer stretch to be at night, not during the day.

A feed-awake-nap series might work (see p144), though keeping a newborn baby awake is sometimes easier said than done. Stimuli such as conversation, massage and new objects to look at are good diversions from sleep. After two or maximum three hours of wakefulness (including a good feed), encourage another nap. Replicate some of the night conditions if you want, though not the bedtime ritual. Either follow your baby's lead as to how long the nap lasts (not beyond three hours). Or look at what evening bedtime you have set and work backwards to encourage naps of a certain duration. For instance, if the evening bedtime is to be 7.30pm, discourage your baby from sleeping past 5pm in the late afternoon.

Encouraging a Good Sleep Pattern

Helping to regulate daytime naps means timing other elements of the day to fit. As noted, encouraging a full feed in between each nap can be an important factor. And if you want to go out, time the journey accordingly: hopefully your baby will sleep in the car, sling or pram to coincide with the ideal nap time.

Sleep Conditioning

Much of the advice compiled so far assumes that there is some difficulty in persuading your baby to settle into a good sleep pattern. However, many babies will start settling within a few weeks and respond well to varying amounts of encouragement and the instigation of ideal conditions for sleep from you. The only catch is that your baby may come to depend on the conditions that you have created as part of the night sleep and nap times.

For instance, if the baby comes to associate sleep with always being in a cot in a darkened room, he may start having difficulty sleeping in any other circumstances. You might find that this kind of conditioning is more of a boon than a problem – it's just when you want be somewhere else that you might get an occasional disturbed night. However, some kinds of sleep conditioning can turn into a problem every single day. Principally, the potential problems are those very ancient methods that we instinctively use to help soothe our babies, namely feeding, rocking and offering sucking comforters...

Feeding-to-Sleep

If you didn't already know it before you had one, you'll soon notice that newborns get sleepy on a full stomach and that sucking is one of their best comforts. So they often fall asleep after feeding. At first, in the very earliest weeks of your child's life outside your womb, when you may be feeling really tired, feeding-to-sleep can be one of your great allies. With relatively little effort on your part, your child will satisfy his or her hunger and quietly drift off to sleep after feeding several times each day. So you might naturally find yourself encouraging this and not trying to move the baby to the cot until fast asleep after feeding.

This is fine for a while, but there will always be times in the early weeks when sleeping doesn't automatically follow feeding even when you want it to. And as the weeks go by, your deliberate use of the ploy of feeding-to-sleep becomes more problematic. The reasons for this may not be obvious at first. But the baby becomes increasingly alert as its brain matures and is able to stay awake even with a full stomach. Feeding-to-sleep then becomes more prolonged. On the other hand, the more you persist with feeding-to-sleep, the more the baby is learning to depend on comfort feeding in order to fall asleep. Feeding-to-sleep then becomes necessary as well as prolonged. This kind of conditioning can start getting in the way of the other methods you might be trying to encourage your baby to sleep better at night, without wanting to feed.

The easiest and most gentle way to avoid this kind of problematic conditioning is to start putting the baby in the cot when he or she is sleepy following a feed, but not yet fully asleep. This may mean unlatching the mouth from your breast once the sucking has slowed right down and risking some fussing and crying. Because of this risk, you might want to start doing the unlatching for daytime naps and after the bedtime ritual, when you have enough energy to handle the fussing. (See the section on how to tell when your baby has taken his fill of milk, p138).

For the time being you might want to continue feeding-to-sleep in the middle of the night when your energy levels are at their lowest and when any liveliness from your baby is most likely to frustrate you. Once your baby starts being happy to fall asleep without having to be fed-to-sleep in the daytime, you may find that the night sleep automatically becomes longer anyway – the baby's dependance on comfort feeding is generally diminished.

Having said that feeding-to-sleep in the middle of the night is probably the easiest solution, the sooner you can start at least shortening the feeds, the better. Another factor with night feeds is that digesting a full feed might be initially sleep-inducing but can actually disturb sleep later on. Adults avoid eating heavy meals just before bedtime for this reason, and don't feel hungry if they wake up in the middle of the night. So generally as soon as your baby starts dropping the link between feeding and sleeping, follow this lead. Don't persist in feeding-to-sleep as your main method for helping to induce sleep – that advice is the concensus of the sleep experts.

ROCKING AND OTHER TEMPORARY COMFORTS

When feeding doesn't work to settle your baby, you will probably instinctively try out the time-honoured methods of cuddling, rocking and patting your baby. As with feeding-to-sleep they're fine, at first. But as soon as you can see a sleep pattern emerging it may be best to ensure that it is not also becoming dependant on anything that requires your presence each time. Cuddling, rocking and patting are bliss, but keep them for playful times of the day or as comforts for crying, not as the usual way to help the baby to sleep. Not after the very earliest weeks, anyhow.

Dummies can also turn into a problem. Until the time that your baby develops sufficient hand coordination to pick the dummy up again (from about four months), you will have to keep going back to put it back in. So try to avoid using them for night and nap times.

Encouraging Your Baby to Fall Asleep and Go Back to Sleep Alone

It's a point worth reiterating, especially because all the sleep experts and most of the gurus, even the baby-centred ones, are in agreement about it. It's for the best if your child can learn how to fall asleep without your intervention.

You may find this an astonishing piece of advice if you are in the earliest weeks with your newborn and finding that stroking, rocking and feeding are the most successful ways of comforting and soothing your child to sleep. Indeed, don't feel that you have to suddenly stop rocking-to-sleep and feeding-to-sleep altogether – both you and your baby need and deserve the comfort of each other's bodies. Just bear in mind that in weeks to come you might not want these kinds of bodily comforts to have formed an actual part of the sleep conditioning.

The most gentle way in which to avoid these problematic types of sleep conditioning is to transfer the baby to the cot when she is still slightly awake rather than waiting for her to fall soundly asleep while still in your arms. You can start doing this as soon as you want and are certainly advised to when she gets to two or three months old. Let her settle herself in familiar surroundings that will still be reassuringly the same for her when she wakes up again.

This can be easier said than done, though. The reason why you might have already developed the habit of waiting for the baby to fall deeply asleep in your arms before placing her in the cot is because you transferred "too soon" on previous occasions. She may have woken up and been unsettled for a longer period than if you had waited a few more minutes for sleep to deepen. You may be craving for the baby to sleep because you want to get on with something else or go to sleep yourself, and so you don't want to risk inadvertently waking her up again. It's an understandable situation. But consider the long-term implications. If she keeps waking up from a light sleep when being transferred to the cot now, the transfer itself is only going to get more difficult as she gets older and heavier. And, as noted under the feeding-to-sleep section previously, the time that she takes to go to sleep is likely to increase, not decrease.

You might be able to put the sleepy but not-yet-quite-asleep baby in the cot without any fussing or crying taking place. If there is some fussing then you can either leave the baby to see if she settles in a few minutes or you can pick her up again. There's no right or wrong in these kinds of situations. Parents usually just "feel" their way through them. Your interpretation of your own baby's sleep requirements defines the course of each day.

It's important to understand that even once they are settled and "sleeping through", babies never in fact sleep solidly through the whole night. They wake up or half wake up from various sleep cycles, then go back to sleep again. The same is true of adults. You may not remember half waking up in the night to change position, but you did several times over. (This is covered in more detail on p159.) These awakenings make it all the more important that your baby understands the conditions of her sleep. If she can only fall asleep through feeding or rocking in your arms then she will call for you each time she wakes up in the night because she has found herself in a completely different place. This is one of the principal reasons why you might find yourself still doing night feeds long past the time when they are a nutritional necessity.

Sleep expert Richard Ferber compares the sleep conditioning of feeding and rocking to a situation such as if you, as an adult, like to sleep with a pillow. You like pillows and fall asleep much quicker and more comfortably if you have one. But if you woke up in the night to find that someone had nicked the pillow then you would feel disgruntled, you would understandably be unsettled until you were given the pillow back and could comfortably go to sleep again. But when you wake up again the pillow has disappeared again… and so on.

Therefore, you are best off if you provide sleep conditions that will remain constant. The same cot, the same room, the same low lighting and swaddling can all be constants. Feeding, sucking (whether on breast or a dummy that later falls out), rocking, patting etc will not be constants.

If you are taking things gently you can start by encouraging your baby to settle from a sleepy state to a deep sleep without your constant presence and intervention. Once your baby can cope with this without much bother, you could try seeing if she settles herself in the cot from more awake states. The success of this will depend on you being able to perceive when she is tiring but not yet showing obvious sleepiness. Eventually you'll be able to put her in the cot at sleep times when she is still wide awake and she will settle herself without any more intervention from you. Some babies learn how to settle themselves without ever crying; some sometimes cry for a little while; some always cry for a few minutes, then go off to sleep of their own accord.

Sleep Training

What happens if your baby doesn't respond to your gentle encouragements to sleep at certain times? What if the "fussing" at being put to bed persists for more than a minute or so? Do you let the baby continue to cry or do you pick him up again to feed, rock or stimulate with conversation and toys until the crying stops? How many times do you try before giving up?

Well, the answers aren't definitive unless you are willing to follow an extreme principle of either never leaving a baby to cry or always leaving him to cry until he stops of his own accord. Admittedly, both ways are consistent if extreme. There have been influential proponents of the latter in previous decades, and there are some today, notably Penelope Leach, who advocate the former. Although "sleep training" is a term that could describe all the methods described so far, it is usually used in the sense of the "controlled crying" method.

What this means, basically, is that you put the awake baby to bed when he is tiring and it is time for a sleep. If he starts crying you go back and reassure him with your presence, maybe some stroking and kind words but you don't pick him up again and you certainly don't feed, rock-to-sleep etc. You then leave the room again after a minute even if the crying persists. You wait a longer interval – five minutes, say – then go in again to reassure your baby with your presence and also to reassure yourself that the crying is not being caused or exacerbated by any other factor. Stay a minute then leave again and wait for a longer interval, maybe ten minutes. And so on. Eventually the baby stops crying and goes to sleep. The next night you do the same thing. And the night after.

How long might the crying continue until the baby goes to sleep of his own accord? Some settle within five or ten minutes. Some take up to half an hour. A few take even longer. The crying can be horrible and heartbreaking to listen to. But in just a few days the duration of crying might drastically decrease as your baby grasps the idea that, although you will answer his cries, you will not pick him up again. Hopefully in just one or two weeks the baby will settle to sleep on his own with minimal fussing. Once the baby is happy to settle to sleep on his own you can also apply the sleep training to any crying that occurs in the middle of the night. No night feeds after six months, no rocking – just reassurance, kind words and then leaving for increasing intervals.

This kind of sleep training is advised by sleep experts for babies over five or six months old who have not settled into a good sleep pattern. It is popular with many parents nowadays, and some parents actually try it well before six months. The main note of caution is with dropping night feeds (see pp185–187).

There are plenty of people who are appalled by the concept of controlled crying and would never try it on principle, no matter what age the child. They are perhaps worried that the baby could be psychologically damaged by the process. Obviously, no-one likes listening to hellish wailing at bedtime. However, ardent supporters of controlled crying tend to be those who tried it and found that it helped in an almost miraculous way. Their babies started to sleep much better than before and were cheerful when awake, showing no sign of psychological distress. The parents then slept better and were more cheerful. However, some parents have tried this kind of sleep training for many nights in a row without noticing any decrease in crying. They therefore gave up with it. On pp189–194 are some stories about sleep and sleep training.

A Middle-Way Sleep Strategy

Here is a suggested strategy to help both you and your baby get more sleep in line with the baby's natural rate of maturing sleep cycles. It represents a middle-of-the-road approach: a bit baby-led and a bit parent-led. Feel free to adapt things as you see fit – earlier or later than suggested, or not at all.

The Very Earliest Days

The first three or four days after birth will probably not be typical of what will follow in the way of sleep patterns.

Your sleep Depending on what kind of birth you have had, you might either be in a state of adrenaline-sustained excitement, hardly able to sleep through the sheer wonder of having produced a baby, or you might be more conked out or shocked or in a state of trauma than excited. Your sleep will be disturbed both by the baby and, if you are in hospital, by the background noise.

Your baby's sleep Your baby, meanwhile, might spend the first few hours of life outside your womb bright-eyed and bushy-tailed, or might be extremely sleepy for several days, especially if drugs were used for a difficult, prolonged labour. A chaotic hospital environment – clattering trolleys, bright lights, voices and other babies crying – will not stop her falling asleep.

Suggested strategy to get more sleep If you are exhausted, then a midwife might be able to look after your baby so that you can sleep/rest for a longer stretch. Note that the practice in some hospitals of midwives feeding with formula while the mother sleeps is criticised by breastfeeding experts. Research suggests that a single feed of formula to a newborn has the potential to lay the ground for lifelong allergy (perhaps to cow's milk itself); also there is a statistical correlation between early formula-feeding in the maternity unit and women who have totally given up breastfeeding by six weeks. Whether or not you are worried about the increased possibility of allergy with some early formula, try to breastfeed as soon as you can after birth and bear in mind that it is possible to establish breastfeeding even if you miss a few feeds.

A Middle-Way Sleep Strategy

Midwives and paediatricians will probably advise you to let your baby sleep and feed at random in the first few days, unless they spot a problem. For example, a very sleepy baby might be at risk of dehydration – you might be advised to wake up the baby every three hours or so in order to feed.

The Next Few Weeks

Your sleep(lessness) While you may hopefully be blissfully happy at having your new baby, the relentlessness and strangeness of your new role as mother 24 hours a day is likely to drain you physically and mentally. Further physical challenges become apparent – they are not individually as dramatic and debilitating as birth, but they add up to a tremendous strain on your body and mind. Any adrenaline that kept you going in the first few days will wear off, maybe at the same time as your hormones change and your milk comes in, corresponding with the so-called "baby blues" a few days after birth. Broken sleep will confuse your circadian rhythms. The frequent feeding and comforting of your newborn around the clock will be tiring. Any physical residues from labour, such as backache, lochia bleeding, anaemia and especially a caesarian scar will further wear you out. Your sleep deficit grows each day, with various effects – making you feel generally half-dead or at other times sending you to extremes of emotion.

It should be no secret that alongside the triumph of bringing a baby into the world, these weeks may well be the most difficult of your entire life.

Your baby's sleep Your newborn baby does not have any circadian, 24-hour rhythms (see pp160–161) at first. The sleeps will be taken randomly in eight or so bursts over 24 hours, ranging from maybe 20 minutes up to four hours each. Altogether she will be spending more than half her time asleep, and half of that sleep time in dreaming, REM mode. She might involuntarily "startle" during sleep – flinging out her arms and legs uncontrollably.

In between sleeps she will feed, be alert to her surroundings and sometimes, or perhaps often, cry. But, with your help, by the end of the first month she will hopefully be taking a greater proportion of sleep at night, and there should be the beginnings of the circadian rhythms.

Suggested strategy Probably the main thing you need in these inevitably difficult weeks is support from other people. Moral and practical support – help with cooking, shopping, rocking the baby or taking her for a walk – anything that will help you get more rest. If family and friends are not available, at least consider hiring some domestic help with shopping, cooking, cleaning etc.

Sort out any difficulties with breastfeeding – establishing breastfeeding will help with establishing a good sleep pattern in due course. You are probably in the very worst of breastfeeding if the "let-down" reflex is painful and if the baby is feeding more frequently than you feel you can bear. However, if you can hold out, breastfeeding may be much, much easier within a few weeks. If breastfeeding makes you thirsty, drink extra water to counteract dehydration and also because water is ultimately better than caffeine as a pick-me-up. Practice deep relaxation at odd moments during the day (see p157).

As soon as you can, create a different set of conditions for your baby's night-time in contrast to daytime. In particular, darken the baby's room from early evening through to morning (i.e. treat night as 10 to 12 hours for your baby) and try not to take her out of that room between those hours: create a bedtime ritual and do night feeds in a dim light if you can. It's true that she is capable of sleeping through noise, lights and chaos at this stage, but by doing these night-day distinctions consistently you are laying a solid foundation on which she can build her circadian rhythms in the weeks to come.

During the daytime in these early weeks, maybe let your baby drop off to sleep whenever she wants but wake her if she starts to sleep more than three hours in a row. Feed her as soon as she wakes up each time, even if she doesn't immediately cry, then try to keep her awake and amused for a while (maybe up to an hour or so) before napping again. A great rhythm to encourage during daytime is a feed-alert-nap series (rather than alert-feed-nap or random feed-nap-feed-alert-feed-nap etc).

Because this is a middle-way strategy, part baby-led, part adult-led, encourage feed-alert-nap when you can, but not too forcefully in the earliest weeks. For instance, if she starts to cry within two hours of the last feed, maybe see if she can be put down or rocked to sleep rather than be fed again so soon. If this doesn't work and she proves difficult to calm, don't resist feeding again if this seems the obvious thing to do. And if your baby naps for just 15 minutes, wakes to feed then seems sleepy again, it may be better to let her nap again immediately without encouraging a period of alertness. Whatever feels better.

At night, by contrast, encourage a sleep-feed-sleep series and always discourage any alertness. Her stomach is probably not big enough yet to take in all the milk she needs during daytime, so she'll genuinely need night feeds at this stage. Don't rush to feed her if you hear her whimper in the night – she might resettle back to sleep on her own. But if she starts crying properly then let her feed in these early weeks. Hopefully she'll drop off to sleep again quickly after feeding, ideally in her own bed or, if you want at this stage, in your arms. But if she is still wide awake after feeding (and maybe starts crying), try swaddling, still in the dim light or darkness, and resettling her in her own bed. Many parents, especially second-timers and beyond, are prepared to listen to a few minutes of crying in the hope that the baby will learn to settle herself.

If she doesn't settle after a night feed and swaddling – just keeps crying – maybe try rocking her to sleep. If this doesn't work then perhaps offer her some more sucking comfort on your breast or a dummy or bring her into bed with you, if you want. These would not be good ploys further down the line, because they encourage problematic sleep associations, but they might be the best and most blissful option for now.

Just avoid getting her up again and distracting her attention with new stimuli in order to stop her crying in the night – this is the last option to take because it immediately confuses the crucial night and day distinction that you are trying to teach.

Other than these strategies, maybe just take each day as it comes during this raw, emotional time. Things WILL get better.

One to Two Months

You Maybe you'll start to feel a bit better in this month as your body recovers from birth and the baby and babycare become more familiar. But broken nights will almost certainly continue, and your baby's crying and feeding may still feel unpredictable and relentless. Some days you might feel relatively strong and energetic, other days dog-tired and listless.

Your baby The non-REM and REM sleep pattern is beginning to form (see pp159–160) regardless of whether you are following a routine or not. She may also start to sleep for a longer stretch – five or seven hours perhaps – once in 24 hours. Although they may not be obvious, circadian rhythms are being set in motion. She is becoming more alert and may start to deliberately fight sleep if there is some interesting distraction. Some days she might also spend a stretch of time inconsolably crying, no matter what you do – the miserable "colic" that's horrible for both child and parent (see pp95–96, 104).

Suggested strategy The night and day distinctions created in the first few weeks might be bearing fruit by now, with your baby taking her longest sleep at night. If you find that the longest period of sleep is happening during the day, try waking her up after three hours. Sleep clinics say that a reversal night-day sleep pattern is relatively easy to coax round the other way.

If you are putting your baby to bed early in the evening you might find that she starts taking a long period of sleep through the early part of the evening, but wakes to feed in the early hours at the time that you want to be asleep. If this is consistently the case, you could try waking her for a sleepy feed at about 10:30pm in the hope that she will adjust the long period of sleep to coincide with yours. Otherwise, hang on for a few more weeks till she starts lengthening the sleep through the whole night.

If you find you are perpetually breastfeeding much more frequently than, say nine or ten times in 24 hours and finding it tiring, consider trying to lengthen the time between feeds (see pp138–139. If you have got into the habit of rocking or feeding her to sleep, start trying to get away from this now or it might become an essential part of sleep conditioning. If she seems colicky (inconsolably upset), especially in the evening, and no amount of feeding, rocking, back rubbing etc seems to help, try swaddling and putting her to bed for the night anyway. She might cry herself to sleep in 15 minutes or so.

Two to Three Months

You Broken nights will probably still occur, and tiredness may still drag you down, but hopefully you'll at least start to have some longer stretches of sleep on an increasingly regular basis.

Your baby The many circadian rhythms continue to develop, the more so if your baby is getting into a good routine for sleeping, feeding and alertness by this stage. The non-REM and REM sleep cycling advances quickly and by three months is exhibiting many of the same characteristics as an adult pattern (see pp158–160). Her involuntary "startles" will probably disappear. However, in between cycles, which take 50 minutes or so, your baby's sleep will lighten and she'll wake up or half wake, wriggle or thrash around. If you're lucky, she'll then go back to sleep again of her own accord without crying. Many babies will suddenly start going for a much longer stretch at night, maybe 8 to 10 hours. We habitually say "sleeping through", but it's important to understand that night sleep is never solid.

Sleep conditioning is really taking hold in your baby's mind, as is her ability to keep herself awake even when tired. Some babies will be continuing to wake and cry several times in the night. Increasingly, this will be more likely due to confusion at awakening from a deep non-REM sleep and problematic sleep conditioning rather than genuine hunger.

Suggested strategy You could start reducing night feeds from now if your baby isn't naturally cutting them out. There are several reasons for this. If you always resolve night disturbances through feeding, you won't be able to guage when

A Middle-Way Sleep Strategy

the disturbances are due to confusion, not hunger. Feeding, and especially feeding-to-sleep after a confused awakening from deep non-REM is regularly cited as a problematic part of sleep conditioning after three months. Your baby's digestive system should now be capable of taking the majority of her food during daytime. (You'll know that your baby's digestive circadian rhythm is maturing when there are fewer poos in the night.) In relation to this, unnecessary night feeds can also inhibit other circadian rhythms from maturing – bit of a vicious circle.

On the other hand, some babies may not be quite ready to start cutting back on night feeds at this age. There's no definitive way of knowing how your baby's digestion is maturing. You could still gingerly try to discourage the night feeds if you're unsure. The gentlest way is to either unhook the mouth from your breast for progressively shorter feeds or to prepare smaller bottles. Decrease over a period of a few days at a time, and see how it goes. Some people offer a bottle of water for night feeds instead, though this can interfere with the milk supply for fully breastfed babies. If you find your breasts becoming unpleasantly full at night, try expressing just before you go to bed.

If you haven't already, this is a good stage to instigate a bedtime ritual at a particular time each evening. A lot of parents are stricter about the timing of bedtime at night than the timing of daytime naps. If this is how you see yourself proceeding, maybe allow a bit more crying at bedtime than you might during the day in the hope that she will learn how to settle herself.

If the daytime feeding pattern is not dovetailing nicely with the daytime naps in a feed-alert-nap series, perhaps more actively coax it that way. Five or six big feeds set around three naps during daytime and just "snacks" in the night (or a deliberate late evening feed) might be an optimum at this age.

Bear in mind that the night sleep might lengthen even more next month, so an early evening bedtime might still be best even if you are being regularly disturbed in the early hours at the moment.

Three to Six Months

You Broken nights should become less of a problem, and both the day and night might take on a predictability to hopefully leave you feeling stronger.

Your baby Three to four months is regularly cited as the time when babies might start sleeping more regularly through most nights and any colic will disappear. Many circadian rhythms – digestion, respiration, immune system cycles etc – have fallen into place around the sleep-wake cycle by the fourth month. The non-REM and REM cycling is complete by the sixth month.

You may see another breakthrough with the length of the night sleep – up to 12 hours is common by the age of six months, with two or three regular naps during daytime. But her sleeping environment may be of paramount importance now: she is no longer capable of sleeping anywhere at any time as she did when newborn and so may be quite unsettled if things don't seem right. She will continue to wake up in the night in between her non-REM and REM sleep cycles. So long as her sleep conditions do not rely on your presence then she will go back to sleep quietly each time. Otherwise, your nights will still be broken with crying, even though she has the potential to "sleep through".

Suggested strategy Once you are beyond the third month cut down then cut out all night feeds, including any deliberate late evening ones, so that they do not interfere with the circadian digestion rhythm. Only rock or feed-to-sleep in exceptional circumstances. If she wakes up crying in the night, wait a few minutes before responding to a cry, then go in to reassure her with kind words and a few strokes perhaps, but give her the opportunity to go back to sleep alone. If she continues to cry, go back in again after a wait of, say, five minutes, reassure, leave, and so on. You may have to go through this process for a few nights in a row. If it doesn't feel right, though, maybe continue with night feeding, rocking etc for a couple more weeks, then try again. Look also at the timing of daytime naps and feeds: two to three naps and four feeds might be an optimum by six months. Really stoke up on feeds during the day to be more confident that night feeds are definitely not needed. She is quite likely to start "sleeping through" of her own accord, without the need for "controlled crying". Hopefully, you'll now start to get magical mornings in which you wake up, fully rested, then leisurely go to greet your smiling, fully rested child...

AFTER THE SIXTH MONTH

You Broken nights should become the exception, not the rule. Sanity is perhaps beginning to prevail again as your own circadian rhythms are repaired.

Your baby The non-REM and REM cycling involves all the same brainwaves as adult sleep. The introduction of solid foods during the day reinforces the circadian digestion rhythm. She is past the main danger age for cot death, so don't worry when she starts rolling onto her front to sleep at night. She might start sucking her thumb or becoming attached to a blanket as a comforter. Such tactile comforts have taken over from the rocking and swaddling of the earlier months to help induce sleep. Unfortunately, sleep disturbances such as night terrors and nightmares are a possibility after this time, though unlikely to be a feature of most nights.

A Middle-Way Sleep Strategy

Suggested strategy Apply the "controlled crying" method of sleep training if your baby is still regularly waking up crying for a feed or to be rocked or cuddled in the night. By now, there's little likelihood that she will start "sleeping through" of her own accord if she is not already because her basic sleep-wake circadian pattern has been "set" to include your intervention and comfort in the night. You either need to "reset" it or resign yourself to regularly broken nights for the next few years until enough language has developed for you to reason with your child that she can get through nights without always needing you.

If your baby usually sleeps through by now but has the odd disturbed night, try extra comforts, cuddles etc, especially if you suspect a nightmare. Many children seem to go through phases when they are generally more clingy and might start to take longer to settle for sleeps after having a phase of going to bed without any fuss. In phases like these you might want to spend more time on the transition from playing to bed, or reintroduce a bit of sleep training – whatever seems appropriate. A sick baby is likely to go out of kilter with sleep, but once the illness has passed you should be able to coax the former sleep rhythm back without too much trouble.

Early Awakenings After the Sixth Month

Some babies get into a good sleep rhythm in all but one thing: they keep waking regularly at the crack of dawn (or before). They haven't automatically lengthened to a 12-hour night sleep by, say, eight months. Unfortunately, there's not much hard advice for this from the sleep experts. It's possible that the final non-REM/REM sleep cycle has become detached from the rest of the cycles. Suspect this if your baby screams for attention at 5.30am, but happily goes back to sleep an hour or so later. Suggestions on how to handle this are much the same as with other night awakenings – try to ignore at first, then try controlled crying.

If your baby wakes very early and is happy to be awake for several hours, then the final sleep cycle detachment is a less likely explanation. You could look at and tinker with the timing of daytime naps instead. For instance, if the baby is taking three daytime naps, try adjusting them to two, and a longer night sleep may follow. To instigate this change, try to keep the baby up and active for a longer time before the first nap is taken. Other suggestions include darkening the room more thoroughly – light is, after all, one of the main external cues that the brain uses to prompt the circadian rhythms. Perhaps the seemingly more obvious option is to put bedtime back. But if bedtime goes back and early morning wakenings still continue – as many parents find – perhaps bring bedtime forward again. Some parents find this cannot be resolved and they just accustom themselves to starting the day earlier than they would like...

Stories About Sleep

Enough of the politics and theories about where babies should sleep and what the sleep experts say. Here are some real stories about how parents cope with sleeplessness and how the sleep pattern changed for them as the weeks and months went by. The first story is the editor's own, in a diary format.

Rosalyn's Story

Two weeks after the birth "Last night I had the first stretch of proper sleep since birth. Two stretches of three hours in a row! That may not sound like much, but I feel a lot better for it. I was literally trembling with exhaustion when I got home from the hospital last weekend. My birth was quite difficult, and I was kept in hospital for more than a week afterwards. People don't believe me when I say I didn't sleep for the whole time I was there, but it's true. I spent a lot of time lying in bed with my eyes closed, but it was never proper sleep – the ward was so noisy and I felt traumatised.

My baby, Minna, has been feeding about 12 to 15 times a day, and sleeps for anything from one to four hours at a time. Ironically, some of her longest stretches of sleep seem to be during the daytime. I count myself lucky because my boyfriend, Mike, is constantly with me and has been doing all the cooking and stuff. I'm blissfully happy for the three of us to be at home together at last, but never imagined that I would feel so weak and shattered."

One month after the birth "Mike and his Mum have sometimes been able to soothe Minna by swaddling and rocking her, so I can rest in another room. I am still so weak that I don't have the energy to carry and rock her myself – I always end up offering a feed to pacify her. She wakes to feed two or three times in the night, but at least now she has reversed to sleep more hours in the night than in the day. Very annoyingly, I have been having a lot of insomnia and often have difficulty dropping off to sleep after feeding her. Overall, I feel better than I did a couple of weeks ago but I'm still really tired and just walking to the local shops wears me out. I think I must be much weaker than the other mums I know, and worry that I'll never feel strong again. I can kind of cope on hardly any sleep by not doing much else apart from feeding the baby and myself, and keeping us clean! I have been taking Minna to bed with me at about 9pm, letting her feed until she drops off to sleep, then transferring her to the moses basket. We bought some sound recordings for babies, including one of ocean waves crashing and a seagull chirping, which I have been playing in the night. The three of us lie in the dark for hours with this echoing around us. My boyfriend and baby fall asleep; I lie awake or perhaps doze on and off.

I felt seriously close to breakdown one day last week – I was shattered following another night of insomnia, and then Minna spent three hours in the afternoon crying, not wanting to feed or sleep. However, that night I had her cradled with me in bed all night and we both slept through for nearly seven hours. The next morning I was quite refreshed (though stiff from being in one position all night, and having had strange dreams of being on a boat with a seagull peering at me!), and Minna seemed happy and content again…"

Eight weeks "I've started to encourage Minna to feed in a more regular pattern, about every three hours in the daytime and evening. She is crying less, which is less exhausting for us. I've started to look at the timing of her sleeps in between feeds as well, but it all went wrong the other evening. She had been soundly asleep from about 7pm and we thought we'd wake her up at 9pm and keep her awake for a couple of hours in the hope that she would sleep better later in the night. But she just started crying and wasn't interested in feeding. We spent about an hour rocking and rocking her back to sleep and totally regretted having woken her in the first place. She still wakes up at least once if not two or three times in the early hours, though I've heard of some babies of the same age who sleep through."

12 weeks "All sorts of things have changed in the last fortnight! We started putting Minna to bed in our room in the dark much earlier in the evening. This was because we had suddenly realised that the overhead spotlights in the lounge might be disturbing her – she kept crying and twisting her head and body round as if to get away from the lights. Also we were craving a bit more of the evening to ourselves. It's not easy eating supper with a baby sleeping on your lap! A few days later we started putting her to sleep at night in her own bedroom. I had known for some weeks that part of my insomnia must be due to a heightened sensitivity to her every movement during the night. I also started to make a bit more of a routine for bedtime: she gets a bath, lullaby, then a final feed in the dark till she falls asleep in my arms. She still wakes up in the night, maybe once, sometimes twice, but we now regard "night" as 12 hours rather than seven hours long."

A Big Chapter About Sleep

14 weeks "There's been another amazing development. We read a book about sleep and learnt that babies naturally wake up and thrash about every few hours. They have to learn how to fall asleep on their own or they might always call for you to help them sleep again. My strategy of always feeding Minna to sleep in the night was probably teaching her to rely on feeding, especially because I was rushing to feed her whenever she was restless.

So we have started "sleep training" – if she wakes up in the early part of the night, I don't offer a feed, but we take turns to go in and reassure her, then leave the room whether she continues to cry or not. In the first few nights this resulted in a lot of crying (maybe half an hour at a time), which was unpleasant. But in just a week there was a remarkable difference. Last night I put her to bed at 7.30pm, with just two minutes of crying. This morning we woke up and could not believe it was 8am, but there was no sound from her room. I felt sick with fear that she had died in the night. But when I went in to her, there she was wide awake and beaming at me! Having read more about sleep, I can now see that my insomnia has probably been due to disruption to my "circadian rhythms", perhaps triggered by the initial stress of birth and maybe made worse by hormones going mad in my body. On the nights of insomnia, I perhaps only go into what's known as Stage II sleep. This is just about enough to get by on, but it's nowhere near as good as the full cycles of sleep that adults need."

Six months "There is a series of ridges on my fingernails, which tell the story of the stress and insomnia of the first three months. But the past three months have been much easier. Not only does Minna sleep for about 12 hours most nights, we also encourage her to take two regular naps during the daytime. She actually sleeps more hours in total now than she did as a newborn (which disproves the books). On the occasions that she has been unsettled and cries – sometimes for a few nights in a row – we go in and out of the room at intervals until she does settle herself. I never feed her in the night or play the ocean waves anymore. She learnt how to roll over at four months. I worried about her sleeping on her front, but there is no way of stopping her. Keeping the blanket on her is also impossible, so we have turned up the heating a notch to compensate. Recently she learnt how to pull herself to standing in the cot, but doesn't know how to sit down again. This has caused some disruption during the night, as we have to go and lie her back down."

Minna and Rosalyn share a blissful daytime nap together at six months.

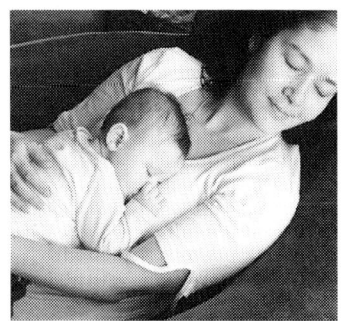

18 months "Insomnia is very rare for me now. Minna still generally sleeps 12 to 13 hours at night, with two naps during the day – I would never have believed she would turn into such a good sleeper! There have been phases when she has been unsettled for a few days in a row – on the occasions when she has been ill or if we have disrupted her normal routine by travelling, when she becomes more "clingy" for a week afterwards. But we have never had to do the sleep training to the extent as at three months.

We have noticed that her second nap has been creeping further back over the last few months, so we are just beginning to try her out with one long nap during the day. She also has nightmares sometimes, when she suddenly starts wailing but is still half asleep. She might go back to sleep quickly if we just stroke her head; other times she gets confused and takes an hour to resettle. These are the only changes to her sleep in a whole year."

Parents' Anecdotes and Ideas About Sleep

Following a prolonged labour and emergency caesarian, Alice suffered extreme sleep loss in the earliest days. "I'd lost four nights' sleep during labour and birth and then spent three nights in a hospital ward with my, and other, crying babies, so I was pretty tired at the outset of motherhood. Then the hormones wore off and the tiredness got worse… In some ways we were lucky because once our baby went to sleep for the night, he actually slept quite well, only waking for feeds and then settling down again very quickly. However, his idea of bedtime was around 3am for the first week or so. Then gradually it shifted to midnight, then 10pm, then 9pm and now it's before 8pm."

Many parents interviewed seemed to have had a really bad patch of feeling exhausted at about three or four weeks, quite different to the so-called "baby blues", which some books describe for about the fifth day after birth. In Alice's words, "the hardship of parenthood really gets to you around three weeks, when the baby's lack of any sleep pattern, combined with your body's loss of its buoyancy hormones just makes you feel terrible and you can't see the way forward. However, just when you despair, the baby begins to finally fall into some kind of pattern of night-time sleep." The experience of those early weeks had scarred Alice and a year later she was still terrified by the thought of not getting enough sleep.

Justine was interviewed at six months and asked to describe the situation so far with sleep. Ella was a "very thrashing babe" in the early days, and Justine had found that swaddling helped her daytime sleeping. She had instigated a calming bedtime ritual of book, bath, feed fairly early on, and Ella had soon got into the habit of falling back to sleep quickly after night feeds. At six months she was going to bed at 7–7.30pm and would wake quite often in the night, but not for feeding. "We tried sleep training at about five months (letting her cry for a few minutes, then comforting without picking up), but she cried for longer than five minutes for a few nights, which was horrible. We tried again a couple of weeks later, having made a pact with each other not to think we were being cruel, and she fell asleep after two minutes! But it took a long time to get to the stage where she would sleep at night without having to be either breastfed or held."

Vicky feels strongly that children benefit from regular sleep. "In the first couple of months I let my baby sleep whenever he wanted. Then he got into a phase at about eight weeks of not sleeping for maybe six or seven hours at a time during the day, and he would end up screaming his head off. The single most useful piece of advice I had from a health visitor was to actively encourage him to take regular naps and put him to bed at a regular time each night. I have stuck to this ever since."

Birth had been fairly straightforward for Caroline, and she had gone home the next day. She was interviewed at five weeks and said she was finding motherhood tiring, though not exhausting. The only time she had to herself was when her son was asleep. She wanted it to be known that "what you hear about babies being able to sleep through noise is the biggest nonsense – he wakes up with any rustling or the click of the door." At this stage, she was usually breastfeeding the baby until he fell asleep, and finding that she had to wait at least ten minutes until he was in a deep enough sleep to be moved without waking. Sometimes he would sleep for 15 minutes, sometimes for four hours. She had noticed that if she accidentally woke him up after 15 minutes then he wouldn't go back to sleep. "This is why, if he has fallen asleep in the car, I sit in the car until he wakes up." At night, meanwhile, she had tried having him in bed after feeding, "but didn't like smelly possets on the sheet". She was actually sleeping on a mattress on the floor of her baby's room for the time being – "I'm doing all the feeding, so what is the point of my husband being woken up as well?" But she assumed this to be a temporary measure.

Many parents mentioned three to four months as an age when they saw a major breakthrough with sleep. But Eunice claimed said was a matter of luck. Her baby was 14 months old and still waking up at least once a night. "Yes, we have tried sleep training several times, but you cannot let a child continue to cry in the night when you are surrounded by four other flats." She was stoical and said that she and her boyfriend had got used to the nights a long time ago. "We take turns to get up and rub the baby's back until he falls asleep again. If he wakes after 5am then he comes into bed with us. It's not as awful as it sounds. In honesty, you adapt to the broken sleep."

Hilary, a mother of four, has sleep trained each child. "Your baby's personality does have something to do with it, and maybe weight – my heavier ones slept through quicker than the other two. I believe strongly that you can start to accustom the baby to sleep at more sensible hours as soon as you're home from the hospital, but you must understand that it is a gradual process, not overnight. And don't expect your baby just to sleep and eat – he needs to be awake and entertained during the daytime, too. However, you mustn't try to keep your baby up for the whole day because he will get miserable."

On the details of when to put a baby to bed, Valerie had this to say: "For the minimum fuss, you have to put the baby to bed when he is becoming tired, but before he gets over-tired. The amount of time is different for each child, but you know when your baby is becoming tired from what kind of sleep he has had in the past 12 hours and what he has been doing and how long it is since the last nap. If you leave it too long to put your baby for a nap, then he will start crying and getting worked up about feeling tired, which keeps him awake for longer. Some babies are happy to go to sleep, others fight sleep. But just because a baby fights sleep doesn't mean he doesn't need it."

All parents felt they understood their babies' sleep requirements after a few months. A few parents with more than one child said getting into a good sleep rhythm was easier with subsequent babies.

In a closer look at sleep training, a couple of parents were asked to note down the exact timings of sleeps over a few days. Mike made the note below on a day when his baby daughter was about five months. With sleep training, she had got into a good night sleep by that stage – her parents could usually put her into bed awake, leave the room and a few minutes later she would be asleep without crying. But the daytime naps were sometimes still tricky.

"12.25pm Come back from shopping trip with her looking tired, yawning and heavy-lidded. Becomes wide awake as I place her into cot, but she is due a nap, so I decide to leave room. 12.30 I spy through crack in door as she pulls herself to standing in cot. She starts crying. I go back in, lie her down and leave room again, ignoring cries. 12.37 Standing up again and crying forcefully. I go in, cuddle her, she stops crying. I lie her down again. 12.43 Hear crying again. Ignore. 12.52 Go in to find her standing up again, rubbing eyes. Stops crying when I lay her down and stroke her back. I remain for five minutes. 12.57 Cries as soon as I leave room. Ignore. Crying is less forceful than before. It is now 35 minutes from when I first put her down. 1.05 All gone quiet. Asleep?

1.06 No! 1.10 Intermittent crying stops without me going in. 1.11 Go in quietly to check. She is standing up, trying to sleep slumped over edge of cot. I lie her down and watch. She rolls around for half a minute, then sleeps on for more than two hours."

Avoiding Cot Death

The incidence of cot death has fallen dramatically. Since 1991 the numbers of babies dying has reduced by over 70% to the current rate of 0.56 per 1,000. **Jane Hobden** looks at the official advice about what measures to take to help avoid cot death and also a look at why these recommendations are made.

A Closer Look at Cot Death

Great advances have been made in reducing the incidence of cot death, and the risk factor is now just one in 1,785 babies, compared with one in 1,050 before the 1990s. However, it is still the most common cause of death amongst babies under one year. Out of about 750,000 UK births per year, about eight babies die each week of cot death, which is more officially known as sudden infant death syndrome, or SIDS, because it doesn't necessarily always occur in a cot. It can affect any baby, but certain babies are at more risk. For instance, 60% of cot deaths in England and Wales are amongst boys, and 86% occur amongst babies under six months, with a peak at two to three months.

Cot death has no single reason. Most researchers think that there are likely to be a number of different causes. Many of the risk factors for cot death relate to the baby's ability to breathe and body temperature. They include babies sleeping face down, being overheated, being exposed to a smoky environment, low birth weight and premature babies (whose lungs are not sufficiently developed). However, in many cases it is not known precisely how these factors lead to cot death.

Social and economic deprivation is another important risk factor, though, again, the links between deprivation and cot death are not fully understood. Mothers whose babies have died of cot death are more likely to be younger, to have more children, to give birth prematurely, to be smokers on low incomes, and living in crowded, damp accommodation.

Minimising the risk of cot death can be done by taking measures to cut out or decrease the known risk factors. The advice overleaf comes from the Foundation for the Study of Infant Deaths. If you take the precautions mentioned, then you have little to fear (see the editor's note about Dealing With Fears About Cot Death at the end of this section).

Avoiding Cot Death

BEDDING OR SWADDLING LAYERS TO TEMPERATURE
15°C Four layers
18°C Three layers
21°C Two layers
24°C One layer
27°C Sheet only or just in nappy

Place babies on their back to sleep Front sleeping increases the risk of cot death, although it is not known exactly why (suffocation is not the cause of cot death). Side sleeping is not as safe as sleeping on the back. At five or six months, it is normal for babies to roll over and they should not be prevented from doing so. Cot death falls rapidly at this age but babies should still be put on their backs to sleep. Before five or six months, gently turn the baby over if you find them on their front, but do not feel you need to check constantly throughout the night. It is also important to let babies play on their fronts, under supervision, during the day to develop their tummy muscles.

Cut smoking in pregnancy – fathers too Smoking in pregnancy increases the risk of cot death. A woman smoking one to nine cigarettes is increasing the risk of cot death four-fold; if she smokes 20 or more cigarettes a day, she is increasing the risk eight-fold. Research shows that a baby's airways function less efficiently where mothers smoke during pregnancy, and there are differences in patterns of breathing. Another theory is that nicotine increases the action of toxins which are produced by bacteria in the nasal passages of babies who have died from SIDS.

Don't let anyone smoke in the same room as your baby Babies exposed to cigarette smoke after birth are at increased risk of cot death, because it affects their ability to breathe. It is best if nobody smokes in the house, including visitors, and to avoid taking your baby into smoky atmospheres. If you or your partner smoke, sharing a bed with your baby increases the risk of cot death.

Don't let your baby get too hot Young babies do not have the ability to control their temperature, so overheating can be dangerous. They are also more likely to become dehydrated which can lead to other complications. A baby will become overheated if she or he has too much bedding or clothing, or if the room is too hot. Check that your baby is a comfortable temperature by touching their tummy, rather than their hands and feet which may feel cooler. Keep the room at around 18 degrees centigrade (65 degrees fahrenheit) – you could try using a room thermometer to keep an eye on the temperature. All night heating is only necessary in very cold weather. In summer, a baby may only need a sheet. Babies should never sleep with a hot water bottle, or next to a heater or fire, or in direct sunshine. When coming indoors or entering a warm car, remove extra clothing even if it means waking the baby.

Keep your baby's head uncovered Babies whose heads are covered accidentally with bedding are also at increased risk of cot death, because it is likely to cause overheating. To prevent your baby slipping down under the covers, place your baby's feet at the foot of the cot or pram. The covers should reach no higher than the shoulders and should be securely tucked in so they cannot slip above the baby's head. Use sheets and lightweight blankets, but not duvets, quilts or pillows. Cot bumpers can be used.

Don't have your baby in bed with you if you or your partner have recently taken alcohol, or some other form of drug or medication which makes you sleep more heavily. This increases the risk of cot death, probably because the parent is less aware than usual of the baby being in bed with them. However it is unclear exactly why.

If your baby is unwell, seek advice promptly Babies often have minor illnesses, but when you are concerned that there may be a serious illness – for instance, if the baby is pale or floppy, finding it hard to breathe or has a high fever – then seek medical advice quickly.

DEALING WITH FEARS ABOUT COT DEATH

Probably most of us harbour some kind of dread about cot death in the early months with a baby. It's not surprising when you consider all the normal feelings of vulnerability and morbidity that hang around at such a time (see pp205–207). We mentally project scenes in which the baby is injured or dies, and imagine how devastated we would feel. An imagined scenario of cot death is perhaps one of the worst, in the most domestic of settings, where you carefully place your precious baby to sleep peacefully. Some of us buy cots, then barely use them when fear comes to the fore. Ideas about family bed-sharing arise in part from worries about babies succumbing to death when away from us. A slumbering baby's breathing often seems irregular, increasing the fear. And the first time your baby "sleeps through" may trigger a sudden panic in you…

But consider this. Fear of cot death is probably normal – perhaps it's a channelling of other unspoken dark thoughts we might have in the early postpartum period into a fear of something that has a name and is well chronicled. The warnings about cot death have the unfortunate effect of creating fear, but also give us something concrete to do to minimize the risk. In fact, your child is very unlikely to die of cot death. Getting beyond embryonic stage (about a one in three chance of dying *in utero*) was your baby's utmost challenge, followed by the risky hours of birth. So long as you don't smoke, and take care with overheating, then you would perhaps have to give birth to nearly two thousand babies to see one die of cot death. Thinking in terms of comparative risk can help to stop normal fears turning into an unnecessary paranoia about sleep.

LOVE AND TRIUMPH

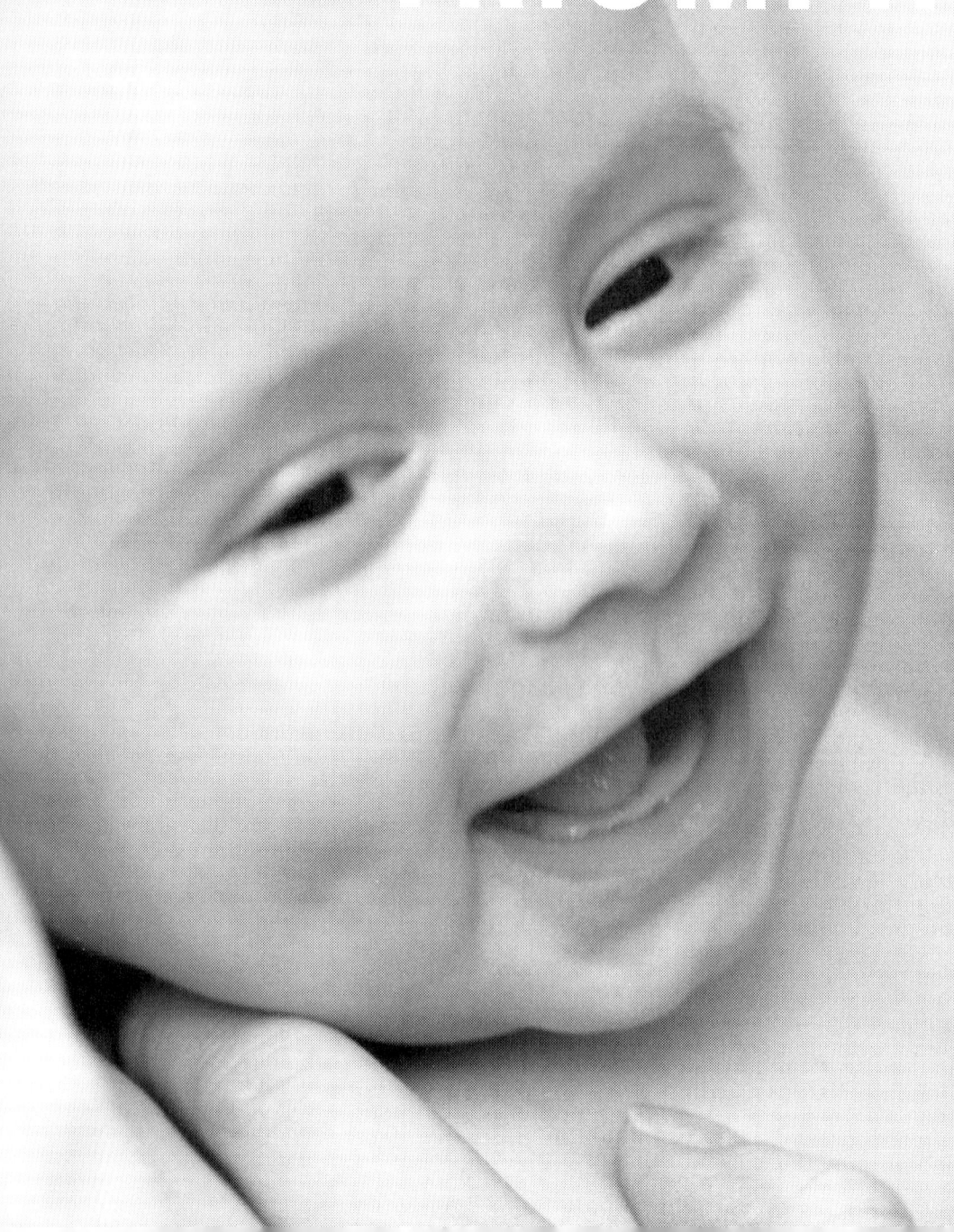

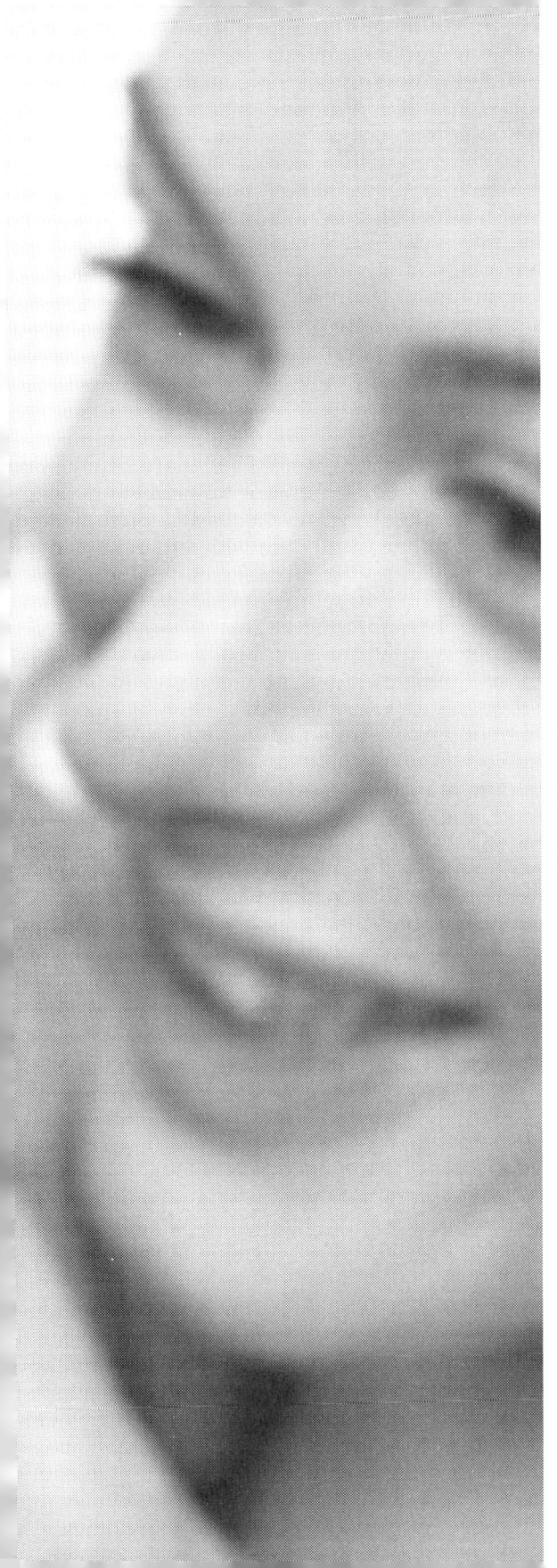

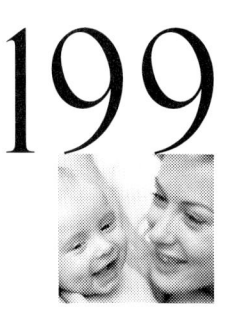

Contents

200 Benign Love

203 Raw Love

208 Deepening Love

BENIGN LOVE

L*ove is a subject rarely tackled in books on pregnancy and childcare. It is generally expected as a natural consequence of having a baby. Yet the complex emotions felt during pregnancy and the beginning of parenthood seem to take a lot of us by surprise.*

LOVING THE BUMP

Pregnancy is both a physical and psychological state, and how it affects us is highly variable. For some women, pregnancy itself is a fulfilling experience; for others it is primarily a time of discomfort and strangeness. Much will depend on extenuating circumstances: other events in your life during pregnancy, how you perceived pregnancy, whether you wanted it at all, for how long you tried to get pregnant, the physical effects of pregnancy etc.

In pregnancy, the love, if felt, is secretive and private. It is one-way, from mother to child, an imaginary love for what you hope will be. After birth, the emotions become fully realised. The baby can bite back, so to speak, feeding your love, rejecting your love, ignoring your love, testing your love and, at times, perhaps reducing your love to tattered shreds. Many new mothers hunger for the swollen-bellied, contented love of pregnancy. This kind of love might be described as "benign". You loved this baby in your body and of your imagination; you fed it with love and it grew to fruition. Outside, the baby's demands suddenly become far more complex, and its instructions immeasurably more vocal and confused. There is a level of control in pregnancy that simply goes out the window after birth. But, with time, the fuller, responsive love of the real baby is bound to be more fulfilling.

The editor asked ten women at different stages of pregnancy what kind of feelings they have towards their unborn babies.

Lizzie was in the first trimester – nine weeks – and happy to declare her love already: "I think of the baby, the size of a strawberry, the tiny, newly formed hands and feet paddling around, secure and happy deep inside me." She had the idea that creating "an aura of love" around the baby might positively influence the child's emotional development. Gail also described a similar idea during her first pregnancy, about "projecting love into the womb". But that baby had sadly miscarried at two months. Now 13 weeks into her second pregnancy, she had tried to suppress feelings of love and excitement through the whole first trimester. "Officially, I started to love the baby yesterday at 10.30am, when we saw it moving on the ultrasound scan".

Other women mentioned the ultrasound as a milestone, to confirm life and perhaps legitimise feelings of attachment. "Everyone says that the scan will be amazing," said Sarah, "but you've got to experience for yourself, seeing your own little baby moving round, its heart beating, so animated and alive – an indescribable joy." Emily was 17 weeks pregnant and said she had been "believing in" the baby for several weeks. "I miscarried before, and there was a miscarriage threat in this pregnancy, too, but that seems to be well over now. I am allowing myself warmer feelings. My boyfriend and I are also now seriously starting to think ahead to what life might be like with a child – for instance, yesterday we were dashing round shopping and doing heavy stuff for the house, and suddenly realised that we wouldn't have been able to do that with a baby to care for."

Feeling movements inside are often mentioned by pregnant women as a significant milestone. The child's presence becomes more obvious, a secret delight for the mother and daily confirmation that it is still alive. Yet a higher level of bonding is not universal among women at this stage of pregnancy. Gerry, 25 weeks pregnant with her second child, had been extremely tired for months. This pregnancy wasn't nearly as thrilling as her first. "It's strange," she said, "because I thought that "the quickening" would be the definite stage when I could relax and start looking forward to the baby. But I've been feeling kicks for about a month now and don't feel any different emotionally. I just want pregnancy to be over with and get on with loving the real baby."

Tanya saw herself as a "glorious fat earth mama". She was preparing to be a single mother and intent for the unborn boy not to suffer from his father being absent. Indeed, her baby already had "love to the power of ten from me and the aunties", as she put it.

Cressie, at 39 weeks of pregnancy, was much more cautious and reflective on the subject of love. "I think I've been in a bit of a cocoon these last few months. It's just dawning on me that I'm in love with the pregnancy, not the baby himself. He will make his entrance soon, and I'm worried about birth defects. What happens if you don't fall in love with your own baby? You can't apply for a divorce! But at the same time, I'm longing to meet him, the faceless passenger." But while Cressie was worrying about what kind of mother she was going to make, Sue was five days overdue with her third child and extremely excited: "It's all there, all the love and anticipation, even third time around. In fact, these last few days are all the more delicious because I know how tremendous and transient this time of life is."

START OF A THREE-WAY RELATIONSHIP

It seems that expectant mothers often feel an exclusive bond with their unborn children, a love that is tied up with physical sensations and self-imagery. This can alter the dynamics in the relationship with the child's father. For the woman, the process of having a baby begins in pregnancy. But for the male partner, birth is more the moment from which life changes. So female and male preparations may be on rather different time scales, and degrees of anticipation and excitement may vary in intensity.

This might sound alarming, but the fact is that, when a baby comes along, the relationship always changes to some degree – from a two-way to three-way relationship. If both partners are prepared to accept and accommodate change, the less likely this will be a problem.

Mike, a father, reflects on this bonding difference in expectant mothers and fathers: "I loved the feel and look of my girlfriend's pregnant belly, but felt less compelled to sit around with my hand pressed against it, waiting for the occasional angular jab. The pregnancy was hers, and that kind of behaviour seemed like a game to pretend it was ours, as if we were going through this together. But the hormones weren't running riot in my body; my bones weren't flexing and my abdomen growing; I couldn't feel the baby as she could." His girlfriend, meanwhile, remembers being irritated at Mike's coolness about the pregnancy. "I thought he was making a miserly rejection of a genuine miracle, a lack of interest in the most momentous time of my life."

Cressie said that going to pregnancy yoga had shown her how much more camaraderie among women there is than men. "After each session we drink tea together, 15 mothers-to-be, and talk about our bodies and our feelings. It's only other pregnant women who can truly empathise. My husband is supportive, but doesn't really comprehend the enormity of it all."

Gail literally feels sorry for men that they can't experience the secret thrills of pregnancy. "My thoughts keep coming back to that old cliché that if men knew what it was to carry and nurture new life, they wouldn't create wars to kill each other." Monica's view was probably the most contentious: "Babies force you into old-fashioned roles, because the way in which you bond with your child is different for women and men. Society reinforces those differences but it doesn't create them. All my friends and I were 30-something career women cohabiting with a "New Man", but now we are nest-builders."

RAW LOVE

From the benign love of pregnancy, birth triggers raw and primitive emotions. We have a way of thinking of parental love as a calm, spiritual love, but the love that awakens with new life in our midst can also be hot, sometimes angry, grasping, painful, tender and passionate. In other words, everything love should be…

LOVE AT FIRST SIGHT?

Some parents profess an immediate love for their children – a kind of love at first sight. Yet, a sudden surge of love for your newly delivered child is, in a sense, still imaginary, in that it is tied up with your expectations and hopes and desires. It is instinctive but irrational – you, as yet, have no idea what this creature is or how you are going to relate to it.

Rosalyn says that she fell in love as soon as her newborn daughter was placed in her arms: "I felt that I recognised her immediately – she was almost exactly as I had dreamed through pregnancy, except I hadn't known for sure that she was going to be a girl and her hair was lighter than I was expecting. Others may have seen a wrinkly baby but I saw her face as a finely sculptured lotus petal. I was babbling, saying "she's perfect, isn't she?", and the hospital staff thought I meant her health and kept reassuring me that she was absolutely fine, but I meant something far more – she seemed so complete and real. I had imagined her and suddenly she was alive, in my arms."

Rosalyn's boyfriend describes a powerful and shocking sense of recognition the moment he saw their child's face, two seconds old and covered in blood.

But many parents – perhaps the majority – do not immediately fall in love with the person they have created and for whom they have a lifelong responsibility. Perhaps the baby looks very different to how they imagined. They feel ambivalent, shocked, even repulsed. But these feelings can rapidly change. Ruth had a traumatic birth (her story is on p40) and says she felt ambivalent towards her newborn daughter at first. "But before long, I was simply astonished by my depth of feeling. I was in the grip of an evolutionary urge to love this creature more than anything else alive, including, shockingly, my partner." Gemma was rather numb, too (see p75). She never felt "detached" from her son, but it did take a little while to bond – a few days. "Since then, the bond has become stronger than I can describe," she says. "I melt every time Liam smiles."

Jo's feelings were ambivalent for a relatively long time. "No, I definitely did not fall in love at first sight, in fact I was revolted. There was some sort of relief that he was alive and appeared to have the various anatomical bits, but otherwise my first thought was one of disgust. His head was mis-shapen, his skin blotchy and wrinkled. Breastfeeding him was also a hideous experience – abandoning that, at two weeks, was the breakthrough. I started to feel happier both with him and myself. Now I am very in love."

Astonishingly, Jo hadn't admitted her bad feelings to anyone at the time, not even her boyfriend. Her view was that lots of mothers are disgusted at first, but don't admit it. "You try to love your child, because it's too tragic if you don't, and eventually you genuinely do."

> *AN ANECDOTE ABOUT WONDER*
> "I still drink in her presence, can never really get enough. Sometimes I feel totally overawed by her – looking down at her sleeping face, much as men have described the feelings of looking at the Earth from the Moon."
> Ruth.

TRIUMPH

Birth is a triumph, no matter what the details. Meeting the person that you created, carried and loved before undergoing the rigours of childbirth involves the most extreme of emotions. A sense of amazement is likely to remain with you through the early weeks, even while you go crazy with sleeplessness and frustration. And perhaps for evermore you will have moments of euphoria in contemplating this wonder of life that you were party to.

Amy felt like a "triumphant bear with her cub" the first day she ventured out of the house with the baby. Another comparison with the animal kingdom was made by Nicky, who was struck with an overwhelming sense of protectiveness within hours of the birth. "A woman turns into a lioness after birth – she is seething with instincts to protect her own child. That feeling actually comes before love. I clutched Daisy for hours and was almost snarling when a doctor came to check her condition."

Some women describe moments of rapture in the early weeks after birth. Eve recalls one evening when Harry was about three weeks old, "rocking him to sleep, gazing into his lovely, serene little face and with tears of happiness rolling down my cheeks. In the thick of all the endless feeding and crying it had struck me again that he was alive and he was mine…"

Jacqui's thoughts were intensely spiritual: "I do think in terms of miracles when I look at my baby. How did everything come together so perfectly from a random mix of sperm and egg? I have sat and wondered about the meaning of life, and where "spirit" comes from, and other religious thoughts." Caroline contemplated with awe the idea of her child's ancestors reaching back through the millennia. She wanted to trace as much family tree on her side and the father's too – history seemed so much more significant than before.

Vulnerability

It appears to be universal that along with loving our children come feelings of vulnerability and a heightened sense of mortality. The worry is for the seemingly fragile creatures we bear and for ourselves, partly because of the ordeal through which we may have come but also because of the responsibility we now hold.

The effect can be, in turn, both empowering and debilitating. Perhaps at times it causes us to fear the world or at least see it as an adversary, something from which we need to protect our children. At other times, however, we may feel more fully part of the world, a greater component of its structure. Parenting can give more of an assured sense of purpose than anything else. As valuable as that is, it can lead to thoughts of insecurity, for the status quo suddenly seems that much more important. Paradoxically, one's own life can seem both crucial and insignificant. Feelings of sacrifice are common, but so are feelings of securing one's stranglehold on life.

The mothers interviewed had some poignant anecdotes about their feelings of vulnerability. These kinds of comments were typical:

"I spend a lot of time worrying about either her being hurt, or something happening to me that results in her being abandoned." (Justine)

"I feel stronger because now I have this tiny little person to protect. Although sometimes, when we go out, I feel quite vulnerable for pretty much the same reason – because I have such a precious baby to look after. I'm still quite hormonal and emotional, which heightens those feelings." (Annette)

"I spend a lot of time just sitting and gazing at my son and grateful that we both made it through birth. On top of that I also feel frightened because he is so innocent and trusts me for everything but I don't entirely trust myself." (Claire)

Siobhan said that she had travelled the world alone and driven down motorways at a hundred miles an hour, but, right now could hardly sleep in case a calamity occurred to her daughter whilst in her care. "She is so helpless, can't even lift her head yet, and you can see her brain pulsating through that soft bit at the top of the skull. My god, she's so fragile that I don't want to take her outside along the pavement. I can't even bear the idea of car fumes wafting over her, and the sight of a lorry charging by brings tears to my eyes."

Feelings of vulnerability can be strong when we are in an unfamiliar environment and surrounded by strangers. This can be the case in hospital, especially a short-staffed, hectic maternity ward. With midwives busy on emergency cases elsewhere, and visiting hours limited to the afternoon, some new mothers are left alone for many hours in the first days with their babies.

Rosalyn felt extremely isolated in hospital, yet she also believes that the emotion of vulnerability can lead to a deeper level of bonding. "On the third morning I left my baby asleep in her cot while I staggered to the toilet at the far end of the ward. I came back to find her gasping and thrashing round, with a great mass of frothy vomit over her blanket and hair. We were both scared by it – in fact, she has never thrown up anything like that ever since. I remember so clearly the way she looked directly in my eyes, terrified and as if to say, "mummy, help." I lifted her to my shoulder and she immediately calmed down. This anecdote might not sound very significant, but for me the moment was a kind of epiphany. For three days, she had been a little creature to be admired – self-contained, keeping herself alive through awesome evolutionary instincts. But suddenly she had become vulnerable, asking for my protection and comfort. I – her mother – was the only one in the world who could help her, and we belonged utterly to each other from that moment onwards."

Morbidness

Terrible events in the news can shake a new parent as never before. Alice was amongst the mothers who had focused on morbid images, above all, the suffering of children. "That photograph in the newspaper of a street in China with a dead baby in the gutter and people just walking past – the dreadful picture has haunted me all week. You feel more appalled by the uncaring and cruel side of human nature when you have your own baby to care for."

Sue's baby, Amber, was three weeks old on the day of the terrorist attack in America. "I sat on the sofa all afternoon breastfeeding and watching the footage of the Twin Towers collapsing over and over again, tears running down my cheeks and feeling almost as if all my family and friends had died there. My innocent child had just been born into a terrible world."

It is not surprising that our feelings of vulnerability can often find themselves in the territory of death. Jacqui found she was sometimes imagining the scenario of attending her baby's funeral, holding the dead child in her arms. She would start crying in reality. Or she would play through an imaginary scene of her own demise, and its effects upon her baby and husband. After upsetting herself for a few minutes, here and there, she would then shake off the mood and strangely feel better for it.

Morbid thoughts can run riot, almost becoming fetishised events. It's hard to rein in such thoughts but, so long as we don't dwell on them endlessly, they needn't be entirely negative, as shown by Jacqui's experience. In essence, such imaginary scenarios are merely serving to confirm our love. As Mike says, "I sometimes think that, if I were to die, imminently, what I couldn't bear, would be the final embrace with my baby. If I knew it were for the last time, I could never hold her long enough or tight enough. Such moments seem poignant – it's an unquenchable desire."

Learning the New Rules of Love

A new love is vulnerable. You want to protect it and are acutely sensitive to each minor rejection or shrug of indifference. As we all know, babies cry a lot in their first few months. Knowing this is normal does little to dispel the feelings of frustration and sometimes anger when we are unable to offer succour enough for our babies to be content and happy again. In the first few months, you may be insanely happy to have your baby, but this may not always be enough to sustain you when times are hard. It isn't always easy to love a baby who is effectively terrorising you day and night. We, too, can feel the sting of their rejection. But this is to imbue a baby's actions with levels of complexity and sophistication beyond their scope. We want their smiles to be genuine signs of affection and imagine their cries as the voice of abject misery rather than the primitive beginnings of language and expression.

David feels powerless in the face of his daughter's emotional swings. "Sometimes I'll be rolling around with Lola on the bed and she's squealing with delight. Then she suddenly gets bored. Her little face screws up and I'm immediately desperate to try and make her happy again. Perhaps it's ridiculous to be controlled by a baby in this way, but this has been the way we have related through the whole of the first year together."

Several parents mentioned colic as a trigger for rage both at their beloved child and with themselves. Maria's son, Callum, became colicky at two weeks of age. "Up to that day, he had been easy to comfort with feeding and cuddles, and I felt that we had "bonded". Then, after hours of him crying, I started crying too. What is the point of hugging and singing to your baby when he just twists away from you, screaming? But once I knew it was colic, I didn't feel so rejected."

Louise expressed the most ambivalent feelings of all: "Not that I would ever do it, but I understand how mothers who throw their babies out of the window feel. I learnt within the first month that it's possible to love and hate your baby at the same time. I love him and would die for him, but sometimes I feel like he has stolen every last atom of my life."

DEEPENING LOVE

*O*ut of your raw emotions towards the screwed up, livid alien set before you at birth, a relationship with your offspring develops and takes on a greater sense of reality. The love deepens, strengthens and matures. But it's not necessarily a simple process.

THE BEGINNINGS OF RECIPROCAL LOVE

To love your child and be loved back is perhaps the greatest relationship in the human compass. Why did you decide to have a child, after all? And, as the months roll by, this two-way loving gets better and better. It's likely to manifest itself in ways that are as surprising as the development of your baby's personality – odd moments that catch you off guard, and the little events that sustain you through the hard months following birth. Many parents mention the first smile as being a moment of heart-melting joy, but equally other peaceful times together can make all of the sleepless nights worthwhile.

Justine's description of the way love has unfolded in the first six months is a touching example. "Love has definitely grown, for both of us," she writes. "I think of the quiet feeding moments when we gaze adoringly at each other...her first smiles. From the first weeks she would turn her head so I could kiss each cheek in turn, and her first kiss back to me was extraordinary. Being aware of her eyes following me in the early days was special. She also learnt to put her arm around my back when feeding – like a cuddle."

It's hard to strike a balance when talking about life with a young child. Words tend to get polarised into descriptions of arduousness and misery or times of unimaginable bliss. When the editor gave questionnaires to mothers, the category of love was the one least likely to be filled in, whereas most wrote something about labour, breastfeeding and sleep. This is not because the mothers have little love for their babies, but because it can be difficult to describe deep feelings. In reality, having a baby is perhaps less of an emotional rollercoaster than a beguiling and concurrent mix of the highs and lows. The emotions don't necessarily rise and fall on a linear course; the heartache and the heartwarming more often get inextricably bound in a torrent of emotion. This can be ecstatic, but it also can be hugely draining and highly stressful. Perhaps the best way to convey this is to break down some of the emotions and factors at work – such as possessiveness, sensuousness, communication and the changing perception of life. When the editor asked some parents about these elements in their love, there was suddenly a much greater response.

Possessive Love and Jealousy

A feeling of ownership over your own baby might begin when you are pregnant. Mixed up with your concept of love and getting to know your baby's movements in the womb, it is another benign kind of emotion at that stage.

In the first days following birth you may not necessarily have a vast sense that you and your baby belong to each other. In fact, quite the opposite can occur. Some new mothers describe a sense of disbelief in the earliest days to realise that this baby is their own, and that the world at large expects them to be together. On the hospital ward, for instance, you might compare your own child unfavourably to others around, and be reluctant to take the initiative when yours starts to cry. Surrounded by the professionals, you might be just as happy for a midwife to look after the baby as do so yourself, especially if birth has taken all your energy.

Possessiveness may take a while to strike, but when it does, the sheer force and depth to which it goes might be a revelation. Many parents find that it strikes very hard within the first few weeks, at the same time as the duties of 24-hour attentiveness are etching deeply into the psyche. Yet there is likely to be an even greater depth of emotion to come a few more months down the line. The more your child reciprocates your love – starting with first smiles, looking to you and you alone for comfort, then later showing love through actions and language – the deeper possessiveness digs into your soul.

Possessive love is one reason why going back to work varies in difficulty at different stages. The paid work is perhaps easier than the demands of babycare, but the arrangement of paid childcare is a complicating factor in your new love life. It can be hard enough to pass over responsibility to someone else in the first six months, before the two-way love has had much time to develop. But it might prove unexpectedly harder once the reciprocal love and possessiveness have grown between you and your child.

The strength of her possessive emotions took Jacqui by surprise. "Perhaps I was naive, but I had imagined that the hardest thing about going back to work would be finding a trustworthy and affordable childminder in time. In fact, it has been my feelings that I am "abandoning" her that have been the very hardest thing to deal with." In a similar situation, Rosalyn and her boyfriend decided to postpone the nursery idea when their daughter started showing obvious signs of insecurity when away from them. "I want to guard her love for us," says Rosalyn.

Many people regard possessive love as an essential part of parenting. Annette cannot contemplate "handing over" her beloved baby to someone else to look after. Dawn feels the same way and goes further to say that she believes mothers are under too much social pressure to go out and work, when their "real instinct is screaming to stay with the child". But Parminder, who works part-time, believes that feelings of possessiveness must be suppressed to a degree: "At first I thought I must do everything for this child because he is mine and only I know how to look after him properly. Eventually, I realised that we could both be happy with a childcare arrangement. Now I think it is wrong to believe that you ever have full possession of anything, even your own child. In Asia, the child belongs to the extended family, not just the parents. In the West, paid childminders become the extended family."

Jealous love is a by-product of possessiveness. Similar to the way in which you might be jealous if your partner had other lovers, you might feel hurt if your child starts displaying great affection for others. For instance, it's probably fair to say that most of us are very pleased when our babies show affection for grandparents and friends, but would be alarmed if those affections seemed to begin to match, let alone overtake, obvious signs of love for us. Angela had an anecdote to illustrate this: "I was at my cousin's party. My 10-month old son kept crawling over and wanting a cuddle, and I was so proud to be singled out in the crowd – he was showing the world that he loved his mother. But suddenly he started kissing a distant relative who I've never liked, and I was surprised and a bit irritated by that."

Children tend to build up a deep attachment to anyone who regularly cares for them. Parents whose children are regularly in the care of another have to suppress any feelings of angst about the other relationship, or the situation is blown apart. Charlotte is one mother who reluctantly works full-time for the essential income, whilst her toddler goes to a childminder. "The occasions when my daughter has called the other house "home" are hurtful. But I say nothing because she is so obviously happy with the childminder."

Within a year of birth, your child will start to develop the concepts of possessiveness and jealousy, too. This manifests by not wanting to share belongings, especially not with other children. You may well find that you yourself (or another carer) become the main belonging in your child's eyes. The way these feelings are channelled between the parents and the child forms a major dynamic in the relationship. Vicky and Martyn's baby is close to both parents but started being more clingy to his mother when he was eight months old. Among his first words were "don't go" if she so much as left the room. Vicky says "he now gets jealous if he sees me playing with other children. I'm having to find a balance between reassuring him that I am always there for him, whilst also making him understand that I'm not exclusively his – especially because there's another baby on the way. It's a constant struggle each day. But it's also wonderful to be so loved by him."

SENSUOUS LOVE

We tend to separate different kinds of love, certainly making the sexual distinct from the familial or Platonic. But we shouldn't be scared of thinking about love for our children in terms of passion and craving.

Breastfeeding can be the earliest and most obvious example of sensuous love. Jacqui's experience illustrates this very well. "Breastfeeding was glorious for both of us. Our bodies in a warm embrace together, our instincts satisfied – hers for oral pleasure, mine for maternal nurturing. No-one had told me that the flutter you feel in your uterus as the milk lets down is like a tiny orgasm. Each time that she started sucking on a full breast I had a momentary vision of passionate lovemaking. I know this is a relatively taboo subject – perhaps it's the link with sexual passion that puts a lot of people off breastfeeding in the first place. Also, I can now understand how the innocent sensuality of children can be so easily abused, and I feel even more protective over her because of that."

Babies are incredibly sensual creatures. They want to touch and taste the world around them, they want to stare, grab, put fingers in your ears, mouth and nostrils, they pull at nipples and probe belly buttons. And part of that exploration includes their own bodies too. They seek and find stimulation, often touching what will become sexual organs, much to the surprise of parents. It is perfectly natural and entirely innocent. They are merely on a voyage of discovery.

Rosalyn was shocked when her eight-month-old daughter started stimulating herself. "I was lying down one day letting her wriggle and roll on top of me. After a while it struck me that she was enjoying herself immensely and getting hot and sweaty, and that her movements were all in the groin, rhythmically rubbing. I came to a horrified realisation that she was "frotting" against me and must have been on several occasions previously. I was deeply disturbed by this for ages. I had heard how baby boys can have pleasure with their penises, but nothing relating to baby girls. Then I learnt that it is common, if not inevitable. Since then, I haven't let her frot against me, but she can bounce up and down and blow raspberries on my belly if she wants. In her cot she alternates between sucking her thumb and frotting against her teddy until she falls asleep."

DO MOTHERS BOND MORE NATURALLY THAN FATHERS? This is a debatable point. There are obvious physiological bonds that fathers cannot emulate. However, the editor's view is that the deepest bonding is forged over time, more from hands-on care than the raw instincts triggered by pregnancy and birth. Breastfeeding, when it works well, is a special bond, but not essential for bonding per se.

Inequalities between maternity and paternity leave reinforce the mother's relationship with the child in the early months. With a greater ratio of shared care, however, a father's love for his child can run just as deep as the mother's.

SEEING THE WORLD AFRESH

As babies strive to comprehend and use their senses – from trying to eat stones to losing themselves in the play of light and shadows on surfaces – they teach us again about phenomena and cause us to join with them in a sense of awe at our surroundings. It's no exaggeration to say that their effect can be genuinely profound. David has a lovely anecdote on this theme. "Some of my best times with Lola have been walks in the rain, sheltered by an umbrella. She loves looking up at branches waving in the breeze, and soon began to wave back at the shaking leaves. What a lovely idea, to wave at trees." Jacqui also recalls the early weeks as a time when she relearnt the basics of life. "My baby reminded me that eating is essential as well as pleasurable. To love music and the visual arts are also human qualities. I could calm her hysterics if I put on rhythmic music and dance with her round the flat. I loved watching her eyes looking at things, and the little cooing sounds when I sang her lullabies."

PLAYING AND COMMUNICATING

The expressions, the sounds, the shared looks and the nonsensical babbling create your relationship much more than the menial tasks of babycare. The deepening love obviously comes from time spent together, whether that is playing with toys, reading, looking at pictures, listening to music or any form of communicating. Play between child and adult is not necessarily about mutual enjoyment. You are not going to enjoy in the same way as an infant crawling around on your knees, hiding behind doors, dancing and singing stupidly to TV jingles etc. The enjoyment for you is in the reaction from your baby. Getting close enough to fully witness and sense their thrill at new and favourite experiences, to see the sudden turning points or breakthroughs in your baby's development. It is not overstating the case to say that, over the first year at least, development is often on a daily basis. Minor breakthroughs – flipping over from back to front, pointing, responding to words, chuckles, making sounds, the first attempts to crawl and to walk – all happen rapidly. One day they are not doing these things, the next they are.

Communicating at six months...

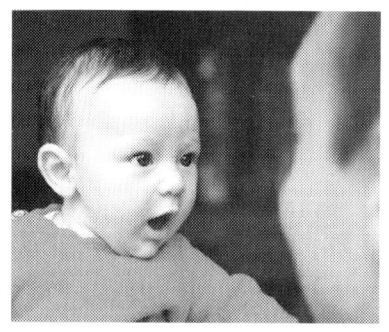

Gemma describes her favourite pastimes with her seven-month-old son as "building towers with blocks for him to knock over, and playing ball together. I love tickling him and throwing him in the air and spinning him round to make him giggle. It's also lovely watching other people with Liam and seeing him make them smile – I'm very proud of him when that happens. Best of all are the times when he tries to imitate my gestures. I look forward to Liam being able to talk to me." Lizzie's baby began initiating hiding and chasing games at five or six months. "I was struck yet again that here was another being, another mind at work, not just imitative but creative too," she writes.

Not surprisingly, all the parents with older babies and toddlers mentioned the emergence of talking as very significant in their deepening relationship. Several said that they were enjoying parenthood much more now that their child had begun to mimic sounds and communicate with words. Richard and Alison were amused by Joey's overnight discovery of the word "door", pronounced inexplicably in a thick Scottish accent. Rosalyn's daughter had just learnt "happy". Jo, who had taken a relatively long time to bond with her son (p204), was overwhelmed when he first said "I love you, mummy," at the age of two.

THE LITTLE IMP IN YOUR HOME

Babies are very sweet, of course, which is why you might have got broody for one in the first place. A child's tiny features are a fusion of its parents' faces, doll-like, rounded and lovable. From birth the eyes dart around, ferociously alive. Everyone wants to embrace the little body, stroke miniature feet and offer a finger to be grasped in a chubby fist. Within a matter of weeks, as the beaming smiles and chuckles begin, the baby takes on the mantle of pure innocence and delight. Peek-a-boo seems to be an instinctive game; blowing raspberries is cause for endless glee.

The onset of clutching and crawling forces you to rearrange household objects. Your baby is now able to shadow you from room to room, pausing along the way for things that have caught the eye: a toy under a chair, a bowl of fruit, fluff on the floor. You get used to the baby's presence at ground level, restlessly moving around. Daily you change your mental calculations about the spans of time in which you dare to relax vigilance – two minutes to visit the toilet while the baby bangs a wooden spoon; ten minutes to prepare lunch while children's TV is on. Standing and walking herald more little nonsenses. The baby seems like a toddler now, in turns childishly mimicking then wilfully ignoring you. Cupboards are ransacked, objects are randomly carried around then either tossed aside or placed with great care in some other receptacle. An innocent kind of mischievousness begins to emerge. The physical presence of your child stumbling around nearby becomes part of your soul.

Hopefully, the evolving relationship between you and your "little imp" will lead your own emotions far more than the introspection in the moments of solitude and insecurity that we all have as parents. Smiles of recognition and whoops of delight sustain you through the hardships of the early months together. And that love just gets deeper and deeper…

THE REST OF LIFE

215

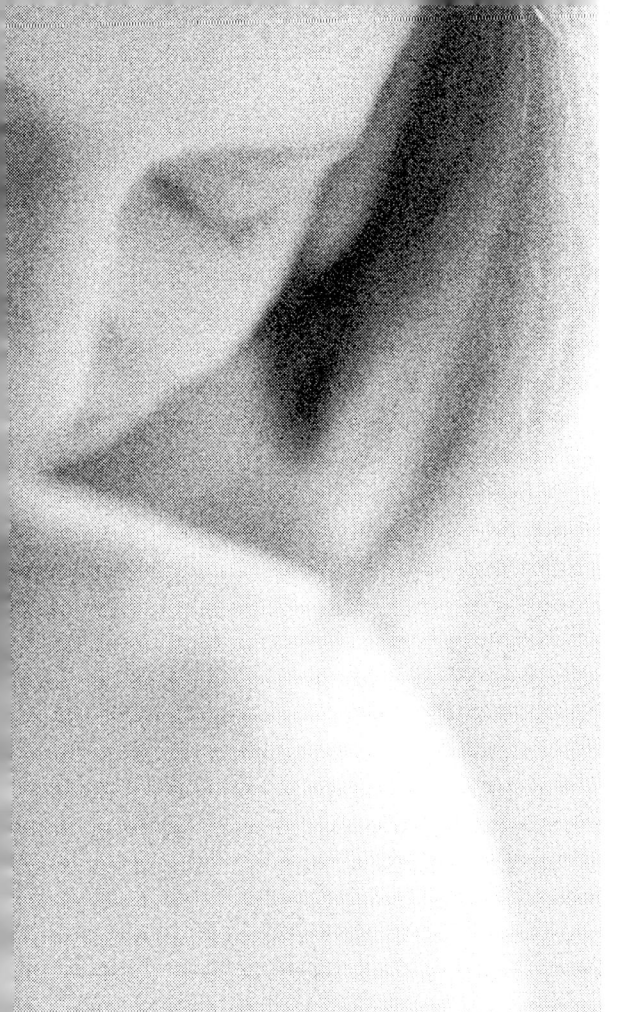

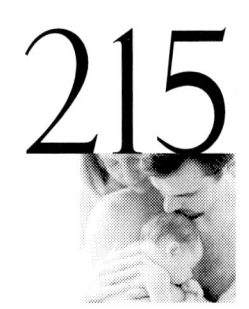

Contents

216 Making Your Baby Official

218 Out and About

220 Combining Work and Parenthood

230 All your Other Relationships

232 Your Sense of Self In All This

Making Your Baby Official

Registering your child's birth is a legal obligation and gives this little person that you created an official identity, with nationality, citizenship and the start of a medical history in the records. Away from the legalities, parents often want their baby to be socially recognised in more spiritual ways.

Making the Birth Official

Many parents regard the signing of the birth certificate at the local town hall as a significant occasion. The process starts with your midwife, who should give you a form stating the location, date and time of your child's birth, which you then take to the local registry office to receive the birth certificate proper. If the mother is not married to the father, then the father has to be present at the signing in order for his name to be put on the certificate. There is no ceremony, and you don't need witnesses as you do for a marriage certificate, but the signing itself can feel like a solemn moment. Once you have the birth certificate you can then apply for a passport for your child, and child benefit.

Christenings and other religious ceremonies are still popular, even with new parents who do not consider themselves very religious. It's not surprising that spiritual thoughts come to the fore when one brings new life into the world. Baby-naming ceremonies are a secular alternative.

Health Checks and Inoculations

Your midwife informs your GP of the birth. The local health clinic will offer a standard number of health checks at various stages of development. Your child gets a booklet into which data from the health checks is recorded. The plotting of weight and growth charts are given great significance in a lot of practices.

Inoculations are another significant part of the health record and, of course, have become one of the hottest topics in recent years. The main controversy – or the one with most media coverage – is the combined MMR (measles, mumps, rubella) jab, introduced in the 1980s. The worry began in 1998 when Dr Andrew Wakefield, then of the Royal Free Hospital in London, suggested there might be a link between the MMR jab and autism and chronic bowel disease. The health authority has since declared that the combined MMR vaccine is safe, but the issue keeps resurfacing in the media. Some parents have decided to have the three inoculations done individually, not available on the NHS, but the health authority says that this is actually less safe than the combined MMR.

At another level of controversy, there is a small body of opinion that any immunizations are potentially harmful, an assault on the baby's immune system. This does not have as much media coverage as the MMR debate, but some practitioners of alternative medicine and sources such as NCT newsletters disseminate information about this theory. Parental worry is not confined to immunizations either. There is even suspicion about injections such as Vitamin K, given just after birth to minimise the risk of haemorrhagic disease. As a result of the worries, nationwide inoculation levels have generally dropped below the point needed for "herd immunity", making epidemic possible.

For the new parent, the weeks following birth are marked by acute senses of vulnerability and protectiveness, and it's not surprising that a lot of us are suspicious of government statements on health given the BSE debacle. At the same time, most of us believe in vaccinations – they wiped out smallpox, after all. The majority do have their babies inoculated, but nowadays many parents go through major worries over the issue in the early months.

Rosalyn (the editor) was one of those parents who agonised over the first set of inoculations: "My boyfriend also worried about whether there might be side-effects, but felt it was a social responsibility to inoculate our own child rather than rely on everyone else to inoculate theirs. It was a nerve-wracking experience to take our precious, trusting two-month-old baby for a jab that we had heard might risk changing her life forever. As it turned out, there was no rash, no fever, nothing. When the time came for MMR, we had stopped worrying so much. We reasoned that in every breath we take are thousands of alien substances that our bodies deal with. To receive a minute, controlled dose of a nasty illness must surely be safer for the immune system than to be bombarded by the real thing. If there was a risk of autism from MMR (and our health visitors assured us that there wasn't at all), it could only be to the order of one in a million or something, whereas the risk of complications arising from contracting measles, including deafness and brain damage, is 1 in 15. In terms of risk factors, the fact that we go cycling with our daughter strapped to a chair on the back of the bike is surely the greatest risk to which we subject her. Anecdotally, I have heard of parents holding "measles parties", so that children who have not been inoculated can "naturally" catch what they believe to be a mild childhood illness. This strikes me as a sign of confusion and ignorance about the real health risks at stake."

Out and About

Getting out of the house with children in tow can be a fraught affair with practical constraints right up until the time that they are happy to be in transit for long periods and understand how to avoid hazards. Parents usually opt for an easier time by keeping outings as local and minimal as possible.

The First Times Out

It's your first opportunity to show the world to your baby and to show off your baby to the world. But preparing to go out can take ages. You need to sort out your own things, the baby's things and the baby itself. Timing between or around feeds will be a factor, no matter how determined you are not to let babycare restrict you. You might be happy enough to breastfeed in public, but you can't breastfeed while driving or as a passenger in a moving car. And while some women astonishingly find a way of breastfeeding their babies in a side-sling while they walk around, this skill is probably beyond most mothers. If you are bottle-feeding, then you will need some way of warming the bottle in order to feed while out. Basically, it's easiest to wait until your baby has fed before going out, then either get back before the next feed is likely to be due or find somewhere to do it at leisure while you are out.

Justine and Mark were excited about their first trips out with their daughter. "We went out with the pram and argued about who gets to push her. I was nervous and dented the pram handle through gripping it so hard!" By contrast, the first trips out for Ruth were nightmarish. She was exhausted after a caesarian and couldn't even lift and carry her daughter. "I had to get a nursing bra and struggled to get from the car to the shop." Like other mothers, she remembers worrying over the baby being too hot or too cold. Julia also found that cars, loud people and dogs seemed so much more menacing than before.

The Equipment

Some of us end up buying a great array of transportation devices for our children. Four parents interviewed had all of the following by the time their baby was a year old: sling, pram, newborn car seat, nine-month car seat, buggy. "I regret the pram" says one parent, "because we only used it a dozen times, which must have worked out as about £15 per time". But for another mother, the pram was essential from the start – she did not have the reserves of strength to carry the baby in a sling. One parent ended up moving out of an upper-floor flat, when the difficulties of having to transport baby, shopping and pushchair in shifts up the stairs became apparent. "I would take the baby up first, then listen to him crying as I went for the pushchair, then the shopping if it hadn't been stolen by the time I got back down."

Few forms of public transport are good for parents with small children. A pram is virtually impossible on a bus and may even be difficult on the train or tube. If you have a folding buggy (not suitable until your child can sit up properly), then learning how to fold it up and gather your other belongings and child to get on and off public transport is another skill to perfect. It may be more environmentally friendly to use public transport, but it is no wonder that many parents prefer to use a car. Three couples interviewed had bought or changed their car when they had a baby.

Trudi had to buy yet another type of pram when she had her second child 19 months after the first. But by then she had got used to the constraints of getting out and about, and knew every easy access point and minor hazard in the neighbourhood.

THE LONG-TERM OUTLOOK

The challenges of getting out seem to go through phases as your child develops. The initial weariness might ease as you get used to the handicapping effects of parenthood. The baby gets heavier but learns head control and how to hold himself upright. He starts to hate having to sit in a vehicle for long periods, but increasingly can move of his own volition. His ability to walk can both help and hinder your manoeuvrability – you don't always have to carry him or constrain him to a pushchair, but he wants to wander off in his own direction, invariably into a pond or the path of a car. There's no other way of dealing with all this but to change the way you do things to suit each phase.

But settling into the new lifestyle and ways of doing things can take months. Hilary recalls how she "desperately kept social engagements" after her first birth. "I was trying to prove to myself that having a baby wasn't as difficult or life-changing as some people had warned. I made a point of going to several parties in the first three weeks after my first birth and didn't admit that I was knackered. I was of the "have baby, will travel" frame of mind before deciding to slow down and go with the flow. Actually, I'm more laid-back now with four children than I was with one. Rather than dashing around, I stick with what's familiar and enjoyable. There'll be time for other stuff in later years."

MEETING OTHER LOCAL PARENTS
Camaraderie from other parents living nearby can make all the difference. Your health visitor should be able to point you in the direction of local playgroups. It's true that your baby won't be playing for some months to come, but such groups are as much for parents as bored children. (They can also be a bit overwhelming at first.) The NCT comes into its own for organising small-scale postnatal groups (see p17). Other ways to forge friendships might be at baby massage classes, "aqua babies" sessions at many swimming pools, and mother-and-baby postnatal yoga classes. Your local health clinic might offer free postnatal workouts – you meet other mums and the exercise sets off "happy" endorphins in your body, too.

Combining Work and Parenthood

To become a working parent is often discussed as something that all women have the right to choose. Yet it is also often viewed in terms of a lack of choice. Whichever it is, involving a third party for childcare can be hard on the emotions, and the practical difficulties of working parenthood can be daunting.

Some Stories About Working Full-Time

Before going into details about the practicalities of combining paid work and parenting, it's worth looking at some contrasting views and stories from parents. The topic of going back to work is, of course, one of the most political issues with having a baby, mainly for the mother.

First of all, two views from mothers who went back to work full-time at the end of their maternity leave. Katie is a solicitor and returned to work after three months. "I had no choice – three months was all I was allowed for maternity leave. It has been very hard, but at least the nanny turned out well and is still with us." Katie's husband, Anthony, is a stockbroker, and she says that they share the parenting fairly equally in the evenings and at the weekend. "It's noticeable that some people are judgemental only about my work arrangements – no-one asks Anthony how he manages both roles. But what is the point of women having a good education if all they do later is wipe up sick and sing nursery rhymes? Working mothers should not be made to feel guilty by society. Just because I work doesn't mean that I love my son any less than a mother who stays at home. In fact, the time that we do spend with him is very intense, quality time. Having said that, I have started to feel lately (at 20 months) that it's very hard to switch between roles, to muster the energy for the evenings."

Justine went back to her job as an immunologist full-time after six months, which included two months' unpaid leave. "I was glad to go back but have always wished that the hours were part-time and I am envious of parents who have more flexibility in their jobs. The nursery is excellent – she loves it, and I have no worries about her being there. My boyfriend works very long hours, so it falls to me to do most of the parenting in the evenings and at weekends, which can be draining. It's quite a difficult life, but not awful."

Stories About Working Part-Time

Going down to part-time hours is an option for some people (see p226). Alice is a marketing consultant and arranged to work for four days per week from when her baby was six months old. "Returning to work was much easier than I had expected. My employer was happy for me to do four days a week, which is not surprising when you consider that I do the same work for less money! My son seems to enjoy being with other young children – they're more amusing than I am to be with. And I enjoy having adult company and being a salary-earning professional again. I had touches of postnatal depression following birth, and am much happier to be a working mother. It's not all plain sailing, though. My boss sometimes expects me to work from home on my day off. I am also aware that my son's needs will change – from a childminder, to a nursery, to a school, with different hours. Then what happens when baby number two arrives? But I guess you just cope with what you have to."

Sally, a qualified architect, had envisaged going back to her old practice for four days a week after maternity leave. "But as soon as Thomas was born, I changed my mind. Trying to fit my old job around looking after Thomas would feel wrong in many ways, and I don't want the stress of attempting it. But I haven't totally given up my career. After a year I found a post teaching architecture for one day a week. I do a swap with a local parent so that we look after each other's child one day and so keep all our earnings. I do feel slightly fraudulent for teaching rather than practising architecture, but I have never once regretted not returning to my old job. If you think about it, people often have career changes throughout a working life of 45 years (from age 20 to 65). So taking a few years of lesser work whilst having children isn't such a long time."

Another solicitor, Helena, developed a similar outlook to Sally. "As the months went by, I realised that going back to my old job would be a huge mistake. I gave up my maternity rights and had a whole year off, which in retrospect I am incredibly relieved about. Now I have just started working three days a week in a different capacity at another firm – in this role I can leave at 5pm whereas in my old job I might still be working at 10pm."

Some parents have found a way of sharing the workload more equally. Claudia and Fred both work, she as a part-time florist, he as a hotel concierge on shifts. Similarly, Rosalyn and Mike are both part-time editors. So far (at 18 months), neither couple has had to involve a third party as carer for their child.

Stories about Misery with Working

The stories related so far are from parents who are relatively happy with their work arrangements. But a lot of women interviewed were not happy at all.

Working arrangements often seem to prove complicated and stressful. Elisabeth now regrets going back to work full-time as a manager in a large IT company when her maternity leave ended 16 weeks after the birth. "I struggled with the juggling act for a year, during which time Bethan had three different childminders (all hopeless) and endless gastro-enteritis, fevers, cystitis and rashes. It was, frankly, awful, yet I kept thinking "life must get easier soon". Then I was made redundant and had a small pay-off. I stayed at home while looking for another job – my husband was encouraging me to cut down to part-time, and I was happier with that idea. I had just found a job when I got pregnant again, so I wasn't sure whether to start the job and in the end didn't. That was two years ago, and I haven't worked since – the cost of childcare for two children doesn't make it worthwhile. I do feel a bit trapped and sometimes get angry about the lack of options, but I am also much happier than I was in the first year. I look back and cannot believe what a mess it was, and why we tried to do it, and I feel that I missed a big part of Bethan's babyhood."

Lisa went back to work full-time as an insurance loss adjuster after her maternity leave ended at seven months. "I was dreading it, but my company had offered three months' extra wages as a bonus if I went back after maternity leave, and they also have a subsidised creche in the building, so it seemed stupid not to take this up. But have you ever tried working out petty insurance claims when your baby is taking his first steps with another woman downstairs? After four months I realised that I wasn't getting used to the situation and was going to have a nervous breakdown if it continued. I asked if I could go part-time, was refused, threatened to resign and meant it, then was offered four days a week. I took this, but kept asking for three days (making myself very unpopular). Eventually, personnel arranged for me to go down to three days a week. This has been much easier, and we can just about get by on the money, but I am not happy about working. My mother didn't have to work because my father's salary as a taxi driver paid for a three-bedroom house. Whereas my husband is an engineer, but all his and my earnings together can afford is a two-bedroom place."

At 12 weeks, Becky arranged to go back to her job as a hairdresser for three days a week "through necessity because I am a single mother". Her retired mother started off looking after her son while she worked. "My work pals thought I was weird for going off to the toilet to express milk, and I soon gave that up!" When Owen was ten months old, Becky's mother tragically had a stroke and was disabled. The next few months were very hard for Becky. "I found a local nursery that could take my son at short notice, but not on the days I needed. The salon owner kicked up a fuss over me wanting to change the days, but agreed in the end when another stylist offered to swap days. Owen cried constantly in the nursery, which was the most awful thing. But after a few more times he got used to it, as everyone said he would. One of my colleagues is a father and very sympathetic, but the others have no idea how hard it is for me. The money is pathetic, too – the nursery now takes about half my wages. It is nice to get away from the baby a bit, but I would prefer not to work at all."

And Some Views from Those Who Don't...

As with the mothers who do work, the ones who don't also have their differing personal views on the subject. Emma knew from before the birth that she definitely did not want to go back to her job as a book editor. "Being a mother is my dream job," she says, "and I don't regret not going back for one moment." Dawn's view is that "mothering has always been the toughest job in the world, but its importance was undermined by the feminist movement and now many ordinary mothers feel their lives are worthless unless they have a career as well. It's a bad state of affairs for the mothers who choose to concentrate on parenting. Instead of being held in high respect for doing a difficult job, we are made to feel inferior. With the money side of things, we survive on a modest income. Of course it would be nice to have more money, but everyone thinks that no matter what they are earning. You mustn't let money or other people's values rule your life. Children need stability and they must come first. It's called sacrifice."

In a somewhat different take on the feminist movement, Monica stated her belief that "post-feminism is all about choice, but in reality women are still forced into a domestic role because they usually bond better with the baby – it's partly biological and partly because fathers don't get enough paternity leave. If we want attitudes to change, then both maternity and paternity leave should be lengthened to at least a year. Then women won't feel pressurised to go back to work before they are ready, and fathers will take on more responsibility for childcare. I was a teacher and will teach again one day. In the meantime, I have bowed to my biological urges to protect my chicks."

Vicky says, "Of my circle of friends, I am one of the few who stays at home the whole time. That wasn't necessarily a particular decision at first, but since having our first child, it seemed the best solution by far. Martyn's job as a computer programmer is not stable, but brings in quite a lot of money when he is working. Another thing that has helped our situation is moving from a flat in a cheap part of London to a house in an even cheaper part of the city. I cannot conceive of anyone else looking after Stan, who is now two and, like many little

FIGHTING PREJUDICE
As some of the full-time mothers have pointed out, they have to battle against prejudice from some people who believe they are being unambitious by staying at home with their children. Yet, other work pales in significance beside nurturing a child through the early years. Full-time parents (be they mothers or fathers) should be afforded greater respect by modern society. You are not an underachiever to prioritise parenting, whether you feel this is from sacrifice or not. Many people will hold you in high regard.

boys, in need of constant reassurance and patience. And, with another baby on the way, the idea of doing even part-time work would just be a pointless complication. I now think that the whole issue of women supposedly being able to be mums, have a career, a social life, run a house etc, is something of an upper middle-class myth. From what I have seen, it is incredibly difficult to do all these things successfully without something giving way."

Annette worked as a managing designer until marrying and having her first child at the age of 39. "I do miss some aspects of my old job, but I couldn't hand over my baby to someone else to look after." Claire, meanwhile, said that she would ideally work part-time if the cost of childcare was much lower.

Allowing Time to Adjust

Having covered some contrasting case studies, it's worth taking a closer look at the practicalities. Particularly if you have just become a parent and are not sure how you want to combine paid work and parenting, if at all, then there are several important factors to consider. To become a working parent can be very stressful, but then so can staying at home be frustrating for some.

First of all, bear in mind that it can take at least half a year to adjust to parenthood. The first few months following childbirth are all about shock, tiredness and getting used to this new, helpless person in your life. The memories of your old life and standard of living will still be relatively fresh in your mind at first, and you may find yourself yearning for them on days when the baby cries a lot and you are alone in the house. You might be in a kind of mourning for your old self. Unfortunately, maternity leave in the UK doesn't take this into account. Either you will not have adjusted to parenthood by the time you go back to work, or perhaps you will have just got into the swing of it, with the fog of tiredness lifting, when the period of maternity leave ends.

Having a baby forces a lot of us to reasses the nature of work itself. In the past, paid employment may have seemed to be the natural order of the world. A career ladder doesn't apply to the work of parenthood. If parenting is to be regarded as work, then of course it is one of the hardest forms of work there is. Yet, as a type of employment, childcare is amongst the lowest paid in society. If parenting has any status at all it is the status of sacrifice and moral honour. The reward is not money and prestige but love and pride. If you subscribe to this concept, then to combine parenting with paid employment might be regarded as a kind of dilution of the role and status.

Then there's the important factor about working for satisfaction. Some people are satisfied and fulfilled by parenthood. Some are not. We tend to build up prejudices about the people who feel the opposite to what we feel on this point. But really we should simply accept our own personal feelings about parenting and never mind other people's perceptions. The problem, though, is knowing how much personal satisfaction you are going to derive from it, which may not be obvious in the difficult early months. Many women who go back to work between two and six months say that the work is a doddle, or feels like a holiday, compared to babycare. But the babycare may be about to get easier and more rewarding, whereas combining paid work and parenting could ultimately be the much harder, more stressful and least rewarding option...

Another new factor to consider is that whereas many co-habiting couples keep their finances separate, parenthood forces you to reassess your life in terms of dependency. As the months go by, parents either grow to be at ease with this changed perception of work and inter-dependency or continue to dislike it, craving more independence.

Again, it's best to allow time to get used to the new situation. In the early months, it can feel that there has been a huge drop in income, which you need to claw back. But think about the situation in a broader context. No matter which way you swing things (working or not working), you will almost certainly be living on a reduced salary for several years to come. Once you have accepted this notion, more options may become apparent.

LOOKING AT FINANCES

Few parents-to-be sit down with a calculator and that's probably a good thing – how many of us would exist if financial considerations were always the priority in life? But if you do, you will find that maternity pay is not worth much. Some mothers feel that they have no choice but to go back to work within a few months of birth for financial reasons. Thus they go back as soon as formal maternity leave ends, whether that is at three, four or seven months.

This may sound like a clear-cut decision to take, but it isn't necessarily. One of the most obvious factors that you have to weigh up when deciding whether to go back to work is the cost of childcare. In the first year, at least, your baby might need one-on-one care. So you have to be earning enough to cover an acceptable level of income for both yourself and someone else. When your child reaches the age of two, the cost of childcare may go down – carers are allowed to take on more children from that age, potentially decreasing the fee for each one. So unless your income bracket is relatively high, you might argue that you can't afford to go back for two years or more, rather than you can't afford not to. Household expenditure might be another thing to look at. Couples often stretch themselves on mortgages etc when both are in full-time paid employment, then panic when children arrive on the scene. There's no easy answer. You need a

CAN THE FATHER'S JOB BE TOUCHED? Even in this era of greater equality between the sexes, childbirth automatically sets a couple on different tracks. Limited paternity rights mean that mothers have the lion's share of responsibility in the early months. Breastfeeding also puts the onus of care onto the mother. The physical bond might be natural, but as we learn from childbirth itself, Nature is flawed.

Options of shared parenting might seem remote when the mother is nearing the end of maternity leave. But if the mother decides to return to work, this actually suggests an equality with the father which, in turn, raises the question why his own job might now be so sacrosanct. This then opens the realm of possibility that both parents might work part-time...

decent home all the more when you have children, but your means of paying for it reduce – whether you work or not. Many families thus move to a cheaper area within a couple of years of birth.

Standards of living relate as much to lifestyle as income. If you used to spend quite lavishly on eating out, shopping, holidays etc you might find your household finances can still work on a lower income level when you tone down these things. Remember to claim child benefit – it may not be much but it helps cover the cost of nappies and baby clothes. Also check whether you are eligible for the working families' tax credit and income tax relief.

Once a few months have gone by you will probably adjust practically and mentally to the lower income. Once the new family income seems like the norm, any extra you might contemplate from, say, part-time work is helpful, but not an absolute necessity. This is bound to be a more positive way of viewing the situation, whatever your course of action ends up being.

PART-TIME VERSUS FULL-TIME WORK

Part-time work is easier to fit around parenting than full-time work and is easier on the spirit. Taking part-time work brings a bit of financial reward, perhaps as much career satisfaction as full-time employment, and might be perceived as just a minor dilution of the parenting role. You will still have lots of time with your child if you work a few hours each week. It strikes a lot of people as a worthy compromise.

The key is flexibility. Freelance workers may initially be disadvantaged through a lack of maternity rights, but later may have more options. In fact, for both parents to work part-time and share the childcare can be the best situation of all: both will have equal status (or at least less unequal status) in parenting, finances and careers. Unfortunately, few couples have the flexibility to take this option. But perhaps more of us need to push for it to become the norm...

Working full-time is very different. If you work 9–5 or equivalent, you will find yourself getting up at maybe 6.30am, having a whirlwind of activity to get the child fed and off to the carer by, say 8am. After work you will be collecting the child around 5.30pm (8–6 are normal opening hours for nurseries, and they are generally very strict with closing time). Most young children need about 12 hours sleep at night, so bedtime will be 6.30–7pm. This gives you about an hour before and after work with your child, mostly spent on practicalities. Few people find it easy to switch between a work persona and parent persona in the space of an hour. These are the basic facts of working full-time: you will either find the day intolerably complicated and always resent not having more time with your child or you will get used to it and not perceive it as much of a problem.

BECOMING A WORKING MOTHER THROUGH CHOICE
If being permanently tied to the house with your child is sending you crazy, and you need to work for self-esteem, then do so. There's no need to feel guilty – some of us actually relate better to our children if we see less of them and have a career to occupy us as well. The children themselves don't suffer if they are in stable, loving childcare arrangements.

Unfortunately, idealised concepts about motherhood – such as that all women must surely feel fulfilled by motherhood alone – persist to a degree. Therefore, prepare yourself for a certain level of prejudice (or curiosity, at least) from some people, especially older generations, if you choose to work for personal satisfaction.

LOOKING AT TIMING

Going back to work varies in difficulty at different stages after birth. At one or two months (as American women know), going back to work is immensely hard on your body and mind, if not impossible in a practical sense. Childcare may not even be available at such short notice.

At three months your baby might be just starting to settle into a pattern, and the physical residue of birth should have largely faded. However, you are still probably tired and reeling from the tumult, and broken nights might still be continuing. If you go back to work now, you may have to give up or cut back on breastfeeding before your child is onto solids (few women manage to express regularly). Partly depending on where you live in the country, you might have had to arrange childcare within the first weeks of birth, if not before. And you may feel a great wrench to be parted from the baby now.

At four to six months your baby might be sleeping through the night, though a fair number don't. Breastfeeding may seem less of an issue (though the UK recommendation is for a year). Your tiredness might be lifting, so the thought of fitting other things into your life might seem more feasible. The practicalities of going back to employment might be easier by now. On the other hand, the attachments between you and your baby will also have grown.

If you decide not to go back at the end of maternity leave, then timing might be governed by how much influence you want to be in your child's early years. Indeed, this is the crux of the matter for some parents – they want to impart their own life skills and philosophies to their children during the pre-school years, when the rate of learning is at its greatest.

Social interaction can be a factor. From around the age of two, children start to genuinely play more with each other, and most nurseries cater for two-year-olds and up. Therefore this is a stage that some parents go back to part-time or full-time employment. Then again, parent and toddler groups also provide opportunities for social interaction, with you in a position to teach your offspring the kind of social skills you want them to develop. The start of the school years is also regarded as a watershed time by many parents. But bear in mind that school hours and school holidays are incompatible with full-time employment. And yet another important consideration might be the timing of having more children…

INSECURITIES

Many discussions about working parents (it's usually talked about in terms of working mothers) focus on balancing the emotional security of the child with a need to earn money. With regard to the child's emotional security, formal studies offer no definitive answers. On the one hand, there may be some positive

---

HAVING NO CHOICE ABOUT WORKING
Much of this chapter is geared to showing that you might have more options than you think about work. Try to minimise the constraints of employment as far as possible because they can create stress.

However, some of us have little choice about working, whether we want to or not. Lone parents and those whose finances are low might find working to be a hard life but preferable to living solely on state benefits. If this is the case for you, then at least make sure to claim the working families' tax credit. You deserve all the support you can get.

benefit for a child to form a range of attachments from an early age; on the other, it can lead to definite short-term and possible long-term insecurities.

Short-term insecurity will be obvious if your child cries when left with the other person(s). Most parents and carers have a transition period for a few days or weeks to help the child get used to the carer and a different environment. The age of your child when making the transition will also have a bearing. Up to six months or so, there may not be too great a display of insecurity, but after this it would be increasingly likely. A toddler might cry when being dropped off and picked up but appear to be happy for the time in between.

The number of carers involved in the early years, the attentiveness and skills of the carers and the ratio of hours with them are all going to have an effect on your child's emotional development, and it is very hard to quantify the long-term effects, whether positive or detrimental. Only you can decide if the childcare environment and people in it are suitable.

Then there might be your own insecurities to consider. It's natural to have secret worries about your baby in someone else's care, even if you trust the carer implicitly. Such worries will hopefully recede as the weeks go by and you get used to the situation. However, another factor might emerge in its place – insecurity over your baby showing great affection to the carer (see p210). Older babies and toddlers often show favouritism, so be prepared for the possibility of the child being more clingy to the carer than you when you are in the same room. This is not necessarily going to be a long-term displacement of affection, but it's bound to have some kind of impact on your own feelings. According to the ratio of hours the baby is with the carer, you are also going to miss a proportion of your child's physical and intellectual development. Some mothers have mentioned a stab of jealousy when the carer reports developmental milestones.

THE ILLNESS FACTOR

Also factor in illness as an inevitable complication, whatever the childcare arrangement happens to be. When a childminder or nanny gets sick you will have to take time off work to cover. (In a nursery, supply staff can cover for sick colleagues.) If your child mixes with others regularly, episodes of illness are likely to increase – children in nurseries easily catch something or other every few weeks. Usually, caregivers don't mind looking after children with colds, but nothing worse, so you will need to take time off work to look after your ill child. You may have to pay the carer anyway. Your own immune system may unfortunately be lowered, too, if you are finding life stressful, so you might be susceptible to malaise of one kind or another. All this is depressing, but less problematic if work arrangements are flexible.

CHILDCARE OPTIONS
Good-quality childcare is defined by the carer(s) close affinity with your child, in keeping with your own way of parenting. It's not necessarily related to cost. Minimising transportation hassles is important.

• Informal – relatives might do it for love, not money. Some parents join up to look after each other's children part-time.

• Childminder – looks after your child in their own home. Must be registered with the local council.

• Nanny – probably comes to your house. Usually the most expensive option.

• Nursery/creche etc – usually from age two, sometimes younger. Some are subsidised by local authorities; others are private. Waiting lists can be long, especially in London.

Rights and Realities

The UK is about average in the Western world in its range of maternity rights: Scandinavian countries, for instance, offer a year or two off, for fathers, too; the USA trails in with its feeble promise of one month's maternity leave after birth (the same country that recommends breastfeeding for two years).

Maternity rights and benefits are a double-edged sword. On the one hand, they force employers to take a social responsibility. On the other, the conditions of your maternity leave might force you into difficult decision-making at a time when you are already grappling with enormous challenges and emotions. But the framework of official maternity leave must not be the main factor dictating your decision-making. You may have the right to go back to your old job, but don't fall into the trap of believing that you must exercise that right. In some ways, returning to work at the end of maternity leave might appear to be the path of least resistance, especially if you were happy at work and your employer is offering incentives, such as extra maternity pay or a bonus if you return (which might have to be repaid if you don't return, or if you return only to resign within months – an intolerable pressure). But many of us don't really know what we want in the first year, and returning to work full time may be very stressful.

Some of us (probably a small minority) do feel more or less ready to return at the end of maternity leave. If you don't feel ready, though, try discussing the possibility of extended leave or a part-time role with your employer. Remember that the main difficulty for your employer is in finding another flexible worker to cover – statutory maternity pay itself is reclaimed through employer's national insurance. If your employer turns out to be inflexible on all fronts, you are then faced with a sort of choice of allegiance – to your inflexible employer, who you perhaps know better than your own child at this early stage of parenthood, or to your child, who you are just starting to know.

The details of working parenthood are rarely openly discussed – we observe other women either returning to work or not, but don't appreciate the practical difficulties and emotional turmoil until we reach the point of having to work out how or whether to do it ourselves. It nearly always affects the mother more than the father, and, in fact, the majority of British women stay out of employment or take on work in a different capacity after they have had a baby. Basically, your decision should be informed by the way you feel about all the kind of factors mentioned. Yes, there are social pressures and prejudices from many directions, and financial considerations. We all end up feeling differently about working, the same as we all have different experiences and feelings about breastfeeding, sleep and love. Wait till the tumult of the early months has settled, then do what feels best, as far as you can wrangle things...

ALL YOUR OTHER RELATIONSHIPS

This is a large subject to cover in a couple of pages. In fact, it is worthy of a book in itself. There's the relationship with your partner, your family, friends and former colleagues. Once you've had a child, it can seem like the world is divided into parents and non-parents; the sympathetic and unsympathetic.*

YOU AND YOUR PARTNER

Of course, there was, hopefully, a love at the very start of all this, between your partner and you. How will this love be affected by a baby – effectively, a new locus for affection that is at least as passionate as the love you have between you? Common fears are that one will replace the other, or at least cause the former love to lessen. After all, how much love can be spread around? In a sense this is true. The vast amount of time spent caring for a baby leaves far less for your partner. However, set against this is the overriding fact that what you have is the most closely shared creation you could possibly make. And the shared love for your new baby often intensifies the feelings you have for your partner.

A few stories to illustrate this point. As Jacqui says: "I've had more arguments with my husband than ever before. I think we've both felt at times, "I'm the one doing all the work." But I also think we're closer and more honest with each other. The way you love your child and your partner are different. There are not enough words for the different types of love. I spend a lot more time looking after Chloë, but she needs looking after; my husband doesn't – well, not so much anyway. There's just a lot of love in my life right now. I don't feel like it's so directional. Every now and then it strikes me how much I love them both. I wouldn't want to pin it down, it's all just swimming about."

Justine: "We felt even closer and enjoyed watching each other interact with the baby. Sex has been great but often interrupted – it makes us feel like we are in a French farce sometimes! But our relationship has gone through some troubled times since I returned to work full-time."

Ruth: "It's only now, 11 months later, that I'm learning to re-direct affection towards my partner. To begin with, the baby just soaked up all my emotions like a sponge. There just wasn't any more to give my partner and cuddle, let alone anything else! That is quite shocking, and I'm fortunate to have an understanding partner. It's all too clear how some couples come under fatal pressure after a baby. I'm still liable to be a bit lacking in emotional energy, but it's important to make an effort. Your child grows more independent over the years, but your partner is for life (ideally!), so you mustn't forget how to love him."

Hilary: "There's that cliché when the doctor says "take some condoms" at your six-week checkup, and you say "I don't need those because I'm never having sex again". But the way you feel soon changes, or I would not have fallen pregnant again, and again, and again! We are both obsessed with and enchanted by our children, which must be the key. I do have friends whose relationship with the baby's father is in jeopardy. The most common scenario seems to be that the father spends too much time away working or socialising while the mother is left to deal with the hardest job on her own. He ends up feeling alienated because he can't penetrate the mother and baby relationship; she ends up despising him for not being there in her hour of need."

YOU AND YOUR OWN PARENTS

Becoming a parent and having to live up to ideals about parenting makes some of us reasses our own upbringing and relationship with parents. As Caroline says, "I now appreciate the hardships that my parents – mainly my mum – went through to bring up my brothers and me on very little money. They were so young at the time, in their early 20s. I do feel closer to them in some ways, and admire my mum's resilience. But she is infuriating when she tells me I'm not weaning the baby in the right way."

AND OTHERS...

Vicky found that she was seeing much more of the friends she had made on an antenatal class than any others. Sharing experiences with others at roughly the same stage of parenthood can be worth much more than all the books and expert opinion put together. Justine expressed some of this: "There is a definite affinity with other parents, no matter how old their children are. Some friends I hardly see or speak to, others I'm closer to, mainly due to the nature of our friendship pre-pregnancy, e.g. drinking/clubbing buddies I see less of, dinner-party friends I see more of."

Pets, too, might be seen in a different light. Rosalyn was infuriated by the constant miaowing and fighting amongst her formerly beloved cats (baby substitutes) – she was relieved when her daughter finally grew larger and more robust than the cats. Siobhan had no time to walk her dog and persuaded her brother to take the animal away to his house.

THE THREE-WAY RELATIONSHIP
Having a baby can bring a couple closer together, but also the inequalities of responsibility can leave both partners feeling like they have the worse deal. A standard piece of advice from psychologists and other parents is that you need time off from the baby to spend as a couple, and you need to be alone sometimes, too. There may be few windows of opportunity, but even an hour here and there can provide the necessary sparkle. Once your baby settles into a more predictable rhythm (from four to six months, say), you will have more time to yourselves.

Your Sense of Self in All This

How are you doing in the face of tiredness, burning love and the ideals of maternal nurturing and self-sacrifice? It's probably fair to say that a lot of us lose touch with our sense of self in the early months of parenthood. But after the first half year or so, many of us then seem to build a new and positive perspective.

Loss of Self in the Early Months

Before giving birth, we probably all have some kind of ideal in our minds about what kind of parent we want to be, influenced by our own childhood, other parents and cultural concepts of parenthood. Many of us have strong opinions about how or whether at all we want to combine parenthood with work. We might look for reassurances of love and support from the other parent-to-be. And women who are inspired by the principles of natural labour might set themselves the target of having an intervention-free birth.

From the onset of labour, we have to start living up to these hopes and ideals, and it is not surprising if some goals can never be reached, or if some high values have to be compromised. How you perceive yourself as the weeks go by will depend on the level of disparity between ideals and reality, and whether you see yourself as succeeding or failing. It will depend, too, on the level of support you get from other people. Tricky stuff, indeed. Most of us eventually seem to come through feeling battered yet happier for the experience. But it is also perhaps not so surprising that one woman in ten (so it is said) gets postnatal depression.

Consider these anecdotes from women in the early months of motherhood. At first glance, all three were projecting an aura of bliss and happiness. But when the editor scratched the surface a bit and asked a few more questions, the response showed the typical turmoil of the early months.

Maria, speaking five weeks after the birth of her son: "I'm choked up with love for my baby, but I've also been tearful and angry. What I can't get over is the lack of time I have to myself – sometimes not even for eating or having a shower. When he sleeps I have no idea whether he will wake up crying again in 20 minutes or sleep on for three hours. Everyone from my grandmother to the

---

POSTNATAL DEPRESSION
The symptoms of depression are often described as insomnia, loss of appetite, disinterest in appearance, lethargy and tearfulness, which might apply to most new mothers. But real postnatal depression (or a deeper level of it) is associated with a total collapse in self-esteem, a loss of interest in the baby and life generally. It is more likely to be suffered by women who were depressed before the birth or for whom the realities of parenthood are utterly different from their expectations. It might be manifest in the early months or take years to become apparent.

Having more support with childcare may help immensely. Counselling and sometimes drugs might also help, so speak to your health visitor or GP if you become depressed.

man on the bus has made judgemental comments like "his hands are cold, where are his mittens?" I want to say back "where is my sanity"? So I'm a crap mother. My husband is cool about fatherhood, but like most dads he's a weekender, not doing it 24–7."

Annette, at two months: "Everyone warns you what it's going to be like, but you don't really understand until it happens. Basically I feel very, very tired and often emotional. Otherwise, I'm fine."

Louise, at 13 weeks: "I have hardly any energy or enthusiasm for anything, and I cannot understand what motivates women to want to be full-time mothers. All I can hope for is that life will settle down in the end. I am probably a good case study for postnatal depression."

SENSE OF SELF AFTER THE EARLY MONTHS

Many new parents seem to start regaining a perspective after maybe six months, when the baby settles and there's more time to rest. The days take on a new rhythm, and any traumatic memories start to fade. You'll get used to a three-way family dynamic. Going back to work might further define the way you feel – it's an added difficulty for many, but can be a boon to some, too. Perhaps the most positive defining factor is reciprocal love from the baby.

Justine, eight months into motherhood, says: "I love being Ella's Mum. I feel grownup at last (I'm only 35!). However, in the stage between stopping breastfeeding and regaining a bit of a waist I was surprised at how unwomanly I felt, like not a mum and not a desirable female." Louise was re-interviewed at 12 months. Compare what she now says with her feelings at 13 weeks (above): "This has been the hardest year, having the baby, my mother dying and moving house, too. But we are a strong family unit and would like a second child. I felt pathetic for a long time; now I know I am a stronger person."

Rosalyn (the editor) found that her own sense of self changed from the middle of labour onwards. Birth was traumatic, and the first three months of motherhood were exhausting. "Yet I have been in a near-constant state of bliss since my baby came into my life, and for now I am exactly where I want to be."

This book deals with complicated and often difficult issues, but ends on a high note, with a lovely anecdote from Ruth, whose stories can be found in each chapter. At 11 months, she says "My life is immeasurably richer because of Rosa. I just feel privileged to watch a human being grow. My self has been added to, nothing has been lost. I rush home from work, so excited to see her at the nursery. I just hope this feeling lasts. (Till the door-slamming, "I hate you" phase?) For now, though, she's like a little radiant, smiling light…"

FEELING GREAT
In the course of the year in which this book was compiled, eight of the dozens of first-time parents interviewed had conceived again. Many others admitted that they were trying for another child and willing to put themselves through birth and broken nights and complicated practical arrangements once again. So why do we do it? Presumably it has something to do with the children themselves – adorable even during the tantrum-laden toddler years. We bring life into the world and so feel that our own lives are more defined and significant than before. It's an addiction to loving and being loved perhaps…

Index

A

abnormality *see* congenital conditions
active birth *see under* birth
Active Birth Centre 17, 18
AIMS 26
alcohol in pregnancy 10
anaemia 73, 182
anaesthetics 13, 21–23
antenatal classes 15, 16–17, 19
Association of Radical Midwives 26
attachment theories 90–91, 99, 162

B

Baby Milk Action 131
baby naming ceremonies 216
babycare
    basics 78–79
    bathing 78
    behaviour 102–109
    contentious issues 84–91
    gurus 80–83
    history 80
    manuals 19, 81–83
    nappies 78
    safety 79
    see also comforts for newborn, crying, routines, breastfeeding, sleep, weaning
back pain 15, 67
Balaskas, Janet 18
Barker, Robin 81, 102–109, 132
bed-sharing 162–164
Biddulph, Steve 81
birth
    active birth 12, 17, 56
    birth plans 34, 71
    birth politics 11, 28–35
    birth stories 38–51
    books 17–18
    classes about 16–17, 19
    history 28–29
    home birth 12, 13, 26
    pain 52–57
    pain relief 56
    natural birth 17, 29–35, 71
    premature birth 75
    recovery from 66–67, 69
    teachings about 16–19
    water birth 12, 13, 16, 42, 44, 49–50, 71
    see also interventions
Birth Centre, The 14

birth certificate 216
Birth Crisis Network 18
birth defects *see* congenital conditions
Birth to Five manual 83, 113
birthing pools 13
bonding 8, 162, 199–213
books
    babycare 81–83
    breastfeeding 130
    feeding 113
    pregnancy 11, 17–18
Bourne, Gordon 18
Bowlby, Edward 81
breaking the waters 20
breastfeeding 84, 93, 96, 103, 104, 106, 112–151
    breastmilk 122–123
    classes 16–17
    comfort sucking 137–138
    counsellors 15, 130–131
    establishing 141–142, 183
    expressing 145
    feeding on demand 134–137
    how it works 114–119
    low supply 139–141
    night feeds 165–166, 176–177, 185, 187
    politics 124–133
    rhythms 134–151
    stories 120–121, 133, 136, 140, 147, 149–151
Breastfeeding Network 131
burping 95

C

caesarian sections 13, 22–24, 35, 40, 43, 49, 57, 67
childbirth *see* birth
childcare manuals *see* books
circadian rhythms 160–161, 173–176, 182, 187
colic 85, 95–96
comforts for newborn 100–101
congenital conditions 9, 74–75
Continuum Concept 91
contractions 20, 21
consultant-led services 12–15
contractions 52–57
cot death 162–163, 195–197
cots 163–165
cottage hospitals 12
    see also midwife-led services

Index

crying 92–101, 102–103
see also sleep training

D
demand feeding see under feeding
developmental milestones 105–109
digestion 103–109, 123
Domino Scheme 15
Down's Syndrome 74
dummies 100, 177
Dunlop, William 33

E
Edgware Birth Centre 14
emotions
in you 9, 54–55, 60, 61, 71–75, 79, 197, 200–213, 227–228, 230–233
in baby 98–99, 208–213, 227–228
epidurals 13, 21–22, 40, 41, 51, 56, 57
episiotomy 21, 29, 33, 39, 44, 67

F
fear see emotions
feeding 84, 93, 103–109, 172
on demand 134–137
summary for first year 112–113
see also breastfeeding
Ferber, Richard 82, 135
Figes, Kate 28–31
foetus 8
forceps 13, 21, 22, 44, 46, 97
Ford, Gina 82, 87, 88, 101, 135
formula milk 103, 104, 106, 113, 122–123, 125, 129, 147, 181
Forna, Aminatta 83
Foundation for the Study
of Infant Deaths 163, 195
Freely, Maureen 83

G
gas and air 39, 44, 47, 50, 56
GPs 12
Green, Christopher 82
gurus 17–18, 80–83

H
Health Education Authority 10
health visitors 15, 69, 130, 216, 217, 219
high blood pressure 20, 45, 55, 73
Hobden, Jane 16–17, 195–197
Hogg, Tracy 82
home birth 12, 13, 26, 60

hospitals
cottage hospitals 12
lying-in hospitals 29
NHS hospitals 12–13, 25–27, 75
postnatal wards 62–65
private hospitals 14

I
illness in baby 97, 228
independence versus attachment 90–91, 163
Independent Midwives Association 14, 15
independent midwives 13–14
induction 20–21, 30, 39
inoculations 216–217
insomnia 155–156
interventions during labour 20–24
statistics 20, 26
versus natural birth 17, 19, 28–35

J
Jackson, Deborah 83, 91, 167

K
King, Frederick Truby 80, 91
Kitzinger, Sheila 17–18, 29, 32–33

L
La Leche League 130
labour see birth and contractions
Lamaze 29
Leach, Penelope 82, 86, 88, 91, 101
Liedloff, Jean 91
love see emotions

M
massage 17, 96, 219
maternity facilities 12–15, 24–27
maternity nurses 69
meconium 103
medical interventions see interventions
midwives 12–15, 64–65, 69, 130
Domino Scheme 15, 27
independent 13–14
midwife crisis 24–27, 64
midwife-led classes 16, 19
midwife-led services 15
team midwifery 15
miscarriage 8–9, 10
MMR 217
moses basket 163

Index

N
nappies 78, 95
   see also digestion
National Childbirth Trust *see* NCT
National Institute for Clinical Excellence 21
natural birth *see under* birth
NCT 16–17, 18, 19, 25, 51, 83, 131, 219
NHS 12, 13, 14, 25–27, 28, 75, 216–217

O
obstetric physiotherapists 15
obstetrics 28, 33, 34
obstetricians 15
Odent, Michel 18
oxytocin drip 21, 22

P
paediatricians 15, 62–63
pain *see under* birth, back pain
parentcraft 16
pelvic floor muscles 22, 54, 66
perineum 21, 66–67
pethidine 56
politics
    birth politics 28–35
    breastfeeding politics 124–133, 165–166
    pregnancy politics 9–11
    sleep politics 162–167, 165–166
Portland Hospital 14
postnatal depression 92, 127, 232
post-traumatic stress disorder 18, 32, 72, 75
pram 218–219
pre-eclampsia 20, 75
pregnancy 7–35
    books 11, 17–18
    love during 200–202
    pregnancy politics 9–11

R
Read, Grantly-Dick 29
rocking 101, 177
routines 80, 82, 85–90, 107, 135, 157, 166
   see also breastfeeding rhythms
Royal College of Midwives 21, 24
Royal College of Obstetricians and Gynaecologists 32

S
Sears, William 83, 91, 162
SIDS *see* cot death

sleep 84, 94, 154–197
    circadian rhythms 160–161, 173–176
    conditioning 176, 178–179, 185–186
    middle-way strategy 181–188
    night feeds 144–145, 165–166, 176–177, 185, 187
    patterns 102–109, 166, 168–194
    politics 162–167
    stories 167, 189–194
    training 179–180, 187–188, 194
    types of sleep 158–159
sling 218–219
smacking 91
smoking 11, 196
Spock, Benjamin 81, 85, 89
St John and St Elizabeth, Hospital of 14
Stoppard, Miriam 83, 86, 101
stress 63–75
sudden infant death syndrome
   see cot death
swaddling 101, 173, 184

T
talking 99
teething 85, 98
TENS machine 12, 42, 56
trauma 71–75

V
vacuum extraction *see* ventouse
ventouse 13, 21, 22, 40, 97

W
water birth *see under* birth
waters, breaking the 20
weaning 84, 108, 113
Welford, Heather 131
Wessex Maternity Centre 14
What to Expect books 18, 83
wind 95
Winnicott, Donald 81
Wolf, Naomi 83
working 220–229
World Health Organisation 23

Y
yoga 17, 19, 56, 219

Acknowledgements

ABOUT THE EDITOR
Rosalyn Thiro is the editor and main author of *Baby and You*. She has commissioned, edited and produced many guides, including consumer guides for Which? Books, travel guides for Dorling Kindersley (e.g. *Eyewitness Thailand, Japan, Scotland, Top 10 Hong Kong, Tuscany, Las Vegas*), art books, illustrated children's reference books, and leisure and lifestyle guides for Macmillan and other publishers. She had the idea for *Baby and You* shortly after having a child and experiencing for herself the great delights and difficulties of motherhood in the modern world.

THE OTHER MAIN AUTHORS
Robin Barker is Australia's most popular babycare expert (see pp81, 102–109, 132).

Kate Figes is a journalist and author of *Life After Birth* (see pp28–31).

Jane Hobden is a medical writer with a special interest in women's health issues (see pp12–26, 195–197).

Sheila Kitzinger is one of the world's leading experts on birth (see pp17–18, 32–33).

The editor would like to thank independent midwife Andrea Dombrowe (p33) and William Dunlop, President of the Royal College of Obstetricians and Gynaecologists (pp33–34), for their statements on birth politics; NCT breastfeeding counsellor Heather Welford for her statement on breastfeeding politics (pp131–132); and Kate Malik and other breastfeeding experts for their views and comments on the breastfeeding text.

THE PARENTS
More than 50 parents have contributed stories and anecdotes to *Baby and You*. A special thank you goes to the mothers who filled in questionnaires: Jo Cavanagh, Eve Elliott, Annette Foo, Alison Gold, Amy Hearn, Julia Mason, Deborah McGurk, Nisha Patel, Emma Perry, Katie Prince, Dawn Roberts, Charlotte Rundall, Ruth Thorlby, Hilary Trevalyan, Caroline Turner, Justine Younsson.

Thanks to friends and friends of friends who told me their stories in person or through email correspondence: Lizzie Andrews, Claudia Bajerke, Tina Bates, Elisabeth Harding, Emily Hatchwell, Melissa Da Silva, Rhiann Evans, Anja Hewitt, Georgina Matthews, Nicky McBride, Ian Midson, Maria Paulo, Vicky Peel, Sally Richards, Louise Vollner.

A thank you to the pregnant women in my local antenatal yoga class, whose babies have now been safely delivered: Gerry, Tanya, Cressie, Sue, Gail and Monica; to Helena from my antenatal NCT class; to Becky and Lisa; to some parents at playgroups, who offered views and anecdotes on various topics: Ian, Teresa, Diana and Parminder at the Leyton Leisure Lagoon; Claire, David, Stella, Christine, Elaine, Colette, Trudi and Angela at the Highbury Fields One o' Clock Club; Sarah, Eunice, Katie and Valerie at the Waltham Forest Toy Library.

Some names have been changed in the book to protect identities.

CONSULTANT EDITORS
Huge thanks to Michael Ellis (boyfriend, confidant, co-author of the Love chapter and the "world's best daddy"); and to

Acknowledgements

Jane Simmonds and Emma Terry for their editorial insights.

PROFESSIONAL BODIES
The following organisations and institutions offered helpful advice and resources in the compilation of *Baby and You*:

Active Birth Centre
Association for Improvements in
    Maternity Services
Association of Radical Midwives
Centre for Biological Timing (USA)
Foundation for the Study of Infant Deaths
Hackney and Waltham Forest
    Health Visitors
Independent Midwives Association
National Childbirth Trust
Royal College of Midwives
Royal College of Obstetricians
    and Gynaecologists
Sleep Research Centre

The advice, suggestions and views in Baby and You are compiled by the editor and therefore do not necessarily reflect all those of the professional bodies listed.

DESIGN
Many thanks to Stephen Bere for designing the jacket, openers and text styling of the book and for putting up with endless talk about babies.

PICTURE RESEARCH
Ellen Root

PICTURE CREDITS
Placement Key: t = top; tl = top left; c = centre; b = bottom; d = detail
Corbis: Terry Vine 3(4), 58–9; Michael Ellis: 45b, 191b; Tony Foo: 39b, 234–8; 164t; Getty Images: FPG/ Ian McKinnell 240; Stone/Elie Bernager 3(8), 198–9; /Dale Durfee 3(1), /Spike 3(2), 6–7; /Philip and Karen Smith 3(6), 110–111; /Terry Vine 3(5), 76–7; Mother and Baby Picture Library/EMAP: Moose Azim 3(3), 36–7; Ruth Jenkinson 115tl/c/b; Pictor Int'l/ PhotoAlto: 3(9), 214–5; Rex Interstock: RESO/Dr. Snuggle 3(7), 152–3; Science Photo Library: John Greim 101b; King's College School of Medicine 29b; David Nunuk 21b; Horacio Sormani 54b; Rosalyn Thiro: 212b; Justine Younsson: 65b, 93b.
Jacket: Getty Images/Stone/Dale Durfee.